PRAISE FOR *LEANING INTO SHARP POINTS*

"I recommend this book for anyone who is or may become a care-giver. Gentle and supportive, Stan Goldberg's essential book should stay on your nightstand throughout the long process from diagnosis to death. You will turn to it again and again for practical, crucial guidance that you will use immediately, and often. I wish I had had such a guide fifteen years ago when I began caring for my son who passed away."

— Dianne Gray, board member,
Elisabeth Kübler-Ross Foundation, and president,
Hospice and Healthcare Communications

"Caregiving is one of the most noble yet unacknowledged activities in our mobile society. With the breakup of the extended family, we have lost much of our innate ability and knowledge regarding caring for the dying. Stan Goldberg, through keen observation and personal experience, gives the reader valuable insights and practical advice on what to expect and how to survive one of life's most challenging experiences."

— Gloria C. Horsley, PhD, president and founder,
Open to Hope Foundation, and coauthor of
Open to Hope: Inspirational Stories of Healing after Loss

LEANING INTO
SHARP POINTS

ALSO BY STAN GOLDBERG

Books

Lessons for the Living: Stories of Forgiveness, Gratitude, and Courage at the End of Life

Ready to Learn: How to Help Your Preschooler Succeed

Clinical Skills for Speech-Language Pathologists

Clinical Intervention: A Philosophy and Methodology for Clinical Practice

Stuttering Therapy: An Integrated Approach to Theory and Practice

Contributed Chapters

The Best Buddhist Writing 2010

Counseling in Communication Disorders: A Wellness Perspective

LEANING INTO SHARP POINTS

practical guidance and nurturing
support for caregivers

STAN GOLDBERG, PhD

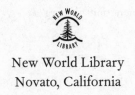

New World Library
Novato, California

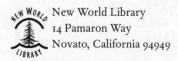

New World Library
14 Pamaron Way
Novato, California 94949

The author's experiences used as examples throughout this book are true, although identifying details such as names and locations have been changed to protect the privacy of others.

Text design by Tona Pearce Myers

Library of Congress Cataloging-in-Publication Data
Goldberg, Stan, date.
 Leaning into sharp points : practical guidance and nurturing support for caregivers / Stan Goldberg.
    p.   cm.
Includes index.
ISBN 978-1-60868-067-2 (pbk.)
 1. Caregivers. 2. Care of the sick. 3. Nurturing behavior. 4. Family relationships. I. Title.
RA645.3.G65 2012
362.1—dc23   2011048954

First printing, March 2012
ISBN 978-1-60868-067-2
Printed in the USA on 100% postconsumer-waste recycled paper

 New World Library is proud to be a Gold Certified Environmentally Responsible Publisher. Publisher certification awarded by Green Press Initiative. www.greenpressinitiative.org

10 9 8 7 6 5 4 3 2 1

Dedicated to all those who have helped me on my journey. I am grateful to my clients, hospice patients, and caregivers for inviting me into their lives. For more than thirty years, your wisdom and compassion shaped my life. Thanks to the Elisabeth Kübler-Ross Foundation for continuing her efforts to make the public aware of the needs of the dying and their caregivers. And also to the agencies and facilities that have allowed me to learn by serving their patients and their family caregivers: Pathways Home Health and Hospice, George Mark Children's House, Zen Hospice Project, Coming Home, Maitri, Gift of Love, Hospice By The Bay, and Vintage of Golden Gate.

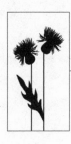

Contents

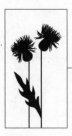

Acknowledgments

Thanks to Kimberley Cameron, my literary agent, for her faith in this project, Georgia Hughes for giving me the honor of publishing with New World Library, and Bonita Hurd for her wonderful editing skills.

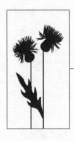

A Note to the Reader

How do I address you, the reader? The use of *you* is intimate but assumes that the reader is right in the thick of caregiving responsibilities. *We* implies that all readers and I share similar experiences, which I know isn't true. *Caregivers* is safe but renders the material less personal. And if this book is anything, it's personal.

Leaning into Sharp Points is for people who now or eventually will ask the question "How do I do this?" and want specific answers directed to them, not to a general caregiver population. I believe most people want to feel as if they are discussing caregiving with a friend who understands what they are experiencing, rather than listening to a lecture about what they should be doing. Within this personal framework, some of the most difficult, frightening, and intimate scenarios of caregiving can be faced. So, if you read *you* or *we* and are offended because I made assumptions about you, I apologize. I allowed the context to tell me how to address you.

WORDS AND STRUCTURE

I use two terms repeatedly: *caregiver* and *loved one*. *Caregiver* is an inclusive term applied to anyone who wants to compassionately serve someone. *Loved one* is the person fortunate enough to have someone who wants to serve his or her needs. They are terms that apply to all of us, if not now, then in the future.

Throughout the book, you'll see the words *serve* and *serving* when I refer to interactions between caregivers and loved ones. I use them instead of *fix* or *help*. According to Rachel Naomi Remen, a physician who has written extensively about end-of-life issues, each term implies very distinct differences in the relationship between a caregiver and a loved one. Fixing occurs when something is broken and needs to be mended. In most caregiving situations, it's more a matter of "accommodating" the consequences of the illness than fixing it. In helping, the person requiring the help is viewed as weak. Although there is most likely weakness, the physical difference often is overgeneralized and applied to the entire person. But when I *serve*, I see the person as intrinsically whole despite the changes the illness has created. A serving relationship is one in which both parties gain.

As I thought about this book, I asked myself the question "If I were writing it for my family, and I were the loved one they were serving, what would I want them to know?" Three things came to mind.

- I'd want them to know what to expect.
- I'd want the information in the book to be practical.
- I'd want them to know what they could do to compassionately serve me.

And that's the information I've tried to supply. Over the years, I've seen so much that's helpful. More than one hundred suggestions for caregiving appear as subheadings throughout the book. All are based on what I've learned from my clients, patients, and their caregivers. What you'll read is what I've seen and heard that provided comfort to loved ones and preserved the sanity of caregivers.

The use of these suggestions also reduced the severity and length of grieving following a loved one's death.

Each chapter stands by itself, so you can use it as a reference guide when a problem arises. Appendix 1 contains a list of websites for national and international organizations where you can obtain much of the practical information caregivers need about specific illnesses and legal and medical issues. Support organizations, services, and groups are listed in appendix 2. Appendix 3 is a list of useful governmental agencies. Appendix 4 is a list of websites where you can obtain information on various end-of-life forms, or the forms themselves. Since there are significantly more pertinent websites than there is available space in the appendices, think of these lists as a sampling of information on caregiving resources. I've also included this same information with clickable links on my website: stangoldbergwriter.com.

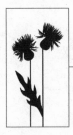

CHAPTER 1

Some Basics

"How do I do this?" he whispered to me. His wife was resting comfortably in the bedroom, and through the open door I heard the rhythmic pulse of an oxygen regulator. One week before, he had enrolled her in the home-based hospice service I volunteered with as a bedside assistant. It was my first visit to their home, and we sat in the living room, where every flat surface was covered with pictures of them embracing each other, their children, and their grandchildren. "We've been married for forty years, but God help me, I don't know what I should be doing," he said.

It's a question asked by millions of people every day when they find themselves, or anticipate finding themselves, thrust into the role of caregiver for someone with a chronic or terminal illness. Their involvement may be continuous, providing physical and emotional care, or sporadic and limited to conversations ranging from pleasantries to final good-byes. While everyone wants to do the right thing, many believe they haven't had enough experience. They look for answers to questions such as the following:

- How do I begin the conversation about how much my loved one has meant and how much he or she will be missed?

- How do I ask for forgiveness for my unskillful acts and words?
- How do I balance my loved one's needs against my own?
- How can I accept abuse from someone to whom I've devoted my life?
- How do I give permission to die to someone who has been a part of my life?

This is not a book of step-by-step directions for caregiving. It's a book of preparation. Preparation for significant others who want to be as helpful as they can to their partners. For adult children who want to repay their aging parents for a lifetime of love. For family and friends who want to do what they can for others who have been an important part of their lives. And for parents who may have the dreadful task of caring for and helping their adult or young children through a chronic or terminal illness. It's also for those in the health care professions who want a deeper understanding of the emotional turmoil that follows caregivers as they serve loved ones and patients preparing to die.

A TRANSFORMATIVE EVENT

We often enter relationships we instinctively know are special, although we may not be able to put a finger on why they are. In many ways, caregiving is that sort of relationship. Some people come to it out of conviction and love; others, from a sense of obligation. It can be a limited experience for family members if there is money to hire full-time caregivers, or a constant experience when finances are scarce or become exhausted. Regardless of why someone becomes a caregiver, the experience will be transformative in both positive and negative ways. There is great potential for enlightenment and tragedy in caregiving, since there is nothing neutral about caring for another human being who can't care for him- or herself.

Accept the Ultimate Gift

We often think of caregiving as a one-way sacrifice. The caregiver gives and the loved one receives. That may define some caregiving situations, but not all. Nick's single mother had been devoted to him her entire life. When he was a child, she cared for him when he was healthy and when he was sick. When he was a young adult, it was her kindness and understanding that carried him through various bouts of addiction. Later, when he fathered a child whom neither he nor the child's mother could care for, it was Nick's mother who stepped in and, even though she was in her fifties, raised her grandchild with all the enthusiasm of a young mother. In her seventies, she hid her cancer from Nick until she no longer could care for herself. After a lifetime of her sacrificing for his benefit, he felt it was time to reciprocate. Since neither Nick nor his mother had funds to hire a caregiver, Nick moved in with her and, for eight months, attended to her physical and emotional needs. After she died, some friends asked how was it possible to provide round-the-clock care for another person for eight months. He said, "She gave the ultimate gift. She allowed me to care for her."

When I leave the bedsides of my hospice patients, I always thank them for the opportunity to visit them. Many don't understand why I'm thanking them. "I'm the one who is grateful to you" is a common response from my patients. Caring for anyone who can't care for himself opens a door to your soul that I don't think is opened by any other activity. The person who allows you to do so is saying, "I'm totally vulnerable and I'm placing myself in your hands." After eight years of caregiving, I'm still learning and, I hope, still growing. You have the same opportunity with your loved one. If you're open to the experience, you'll learn about yourself, death, and, most important, life. But to do that you must be willing to lean into the sharp points of caregiving.

Lean into the Sharp Points

Tibetans say that, to get over the things you fear most — the sharp points of your life — bring them closer instead of pushing them away. It's an idea that many people in Western societies view as counter-intuitive. For example, some try to hide from the sharp points of aging by glossing over them, which has the same degree of success that a new coat of paint on an old car has in stopping the car's engine from sputtering. Some who have lost physical or cognitive abilities grasp at what is gone, doing little more than increasing their suffering. And faced with death — probably the sharpest point of all — we hide from it as if it were a tyrannical schoolteacher coming to discipline us. It is always our choice whether to follow the ancient Tibetan advice.

The poet Rainer Maria Rilke thought bringing the sharp points in life closer was an opportunity for healing. He said our greatest fears are like dragons guarding our hearts. Few dragons are as intimidating or as capable of hiding our wisdom from us as long-term caregiving. Pushing away the sharp points of caregiving is like covering them with a permeable membrane, something porous enough that they emerge at unexpected moments. A smell, word, or sight allows them to resurface. Think about the transformative events in your life. I would guess that most, if not all, involved getting past the dragons. Personal growth doesn't seem to occur when life is pleasant. Few people would say something like: "Yes, I turned my life around sitting on the beach in Kauai being served piña coladas by attentive waitstaff." Just as intense heat and pounding are necessary for creating the highest-quality swords, sharp points are necessary for shaping our lives.

THE DYNAMICS OF CAREGIVING

Considering all the things that can go wrong with our minds and bodies, I'm amazed we can last as long as we do. But when things start going wrong, very wrong, caregivers are often thrust into chaotic situations. Daily, they are often forced to make momentous decisions without much guidance. What was needed yesterday may not be sufficient today. Just when they understand how to care for a loved one, the illness takes an unexpected twist and they're dumbfounded about what to do next. A loved one was grateful for what was done yesterday, but today it's just not good enough. And tomorrow? Will things finally stabilize, or will the roller-coaster ride continue? With chronic and terminal illnesses, nothing stays the same for long. Instead of trying to become comfortable with what you are already doing, it's better to become malleable, ready to move along with the ebb and flow of the situation. Much has been written about the hows, whats, shoulds, and should nots of caregiving. But to clearly understand caregiving, all the peripherals need to be stripped away, leaving its most basic component, *offering compassionate service to someone who can't do things by him- or herself*.

Expect Limited Stability

We can expect celery to always be green, the car next to us at the intersection to stop when the light turns red, and, when purchasing something for sixty cents, to receive forty cents back from a dollar bill. But these assumptions work only when the world in which they exist is stable. Progressive illnesses turn stability on its head. Along with the inevitable changes in loved ones may come changes in their behaviors and personalities, as happened to the husband of a woman I counseled. Her husband was diagnosed with Huntington's disease, and his physician was clear that the illness's progression would be measured in years, if not decades. During the first year after the diagnosis, the husband's caregiving requirements were minimal. He was ambulatory, and medications slowed his involuntary movements. His wife read everything she could find on Huntington's. She understood that, along with the involuntary movements, her husband would experience changes in personality and cognition, and finally, after twenty years of dreadful changes, he would die. During the first year of caregiving, she developed a routine for serving her husband and caring for herself.

Although it wasn't the life this woman wanted or had expected, her love for her husband was strong enough to justify the required changes in her lifestyle. Even though his Huntington's symptoms increased in intensity, her expectations about what she needed to do, and what he was still capable of doing, remained the same. By the third year, unable to adjust to his new changes, she became despondent. The stability that she wanted for herself and her husband never materialized. The lesson I learned from my client was: If you expect stability, you'll be disappointed. Assume that throughout the course of caregiving, the needs of your loved one will continually change, as may his personality and your caregiving responsibilities.

Accept the Difficulty of Change

Change is analogous to a large boulder balanced on a precipice. It looks like it could tumble off the cliff if just a little pressure were applied. But despite your great effort, it won't budge. The weight and inertia of the boulder prevent it from moving. And just as with the boulder, inertia prevents us and our loved ones from changing a behavior that's been with us for a long time. There is a story told of a dog lying on the front porch of a house and moaning loudly. Next to him sat an old man in a rocking chair, impassively whittling a piece of wood. A stranger came by and was amazed by the scene. He walked up to the porch to see what the problem was with the dog.

"Howdy," he said to the old man.

"Howdy," the old man responded, barely looking up from the piece of wood he was carving.

"I was wondering why your hound is yelping."

"He's lying on a nail," the old man said, taking a puff on his corncob pipe.

"How long's he been doing that?" the stranger asked.

"Oh, I reckon about eight hours."

"Eight hours!" the shocked stranger said.

"Yup."

"Well, why doesn't he get off of it?"

The old man stopped whittling, took another puff on his pipe, and stroked his beard as if in deep thought. Then after a moment he looked up at the stranger. "I guess he forgot what it feels like not lying on it."

We are all resistant to change, even when we say we are not. And just like that old hound dog, we fear change's double-edged sword: giving up the known while simultaneously accepting the unknown. Change will be difficult for you and your loved one. Your loved one is moving from independence to dependence, from health to illness, and from being in control to having little of it. You are about to give up significant parts of your life and substitute activities you never would have chosen if your loved one were healthier. Both of you are moving from A to B: from what you were to what you are becoming. It's a rootless psychological state that inevitably causes anxiety. There is discomfort in most transitions, sometimes even fear. You and your loved one will be moving from something you both know to something unknown to either of you. The discomfort can be reduced by holding on a little less tightly to what is familiar. Assume that many things in your and your loved one's "pre-illness" life will lose their permanence.

Be Nimble as the Illness Progresses

We know that in the vast majority of cases where people require extended care, the illnesses are relentless, ultimately ending in the deaths of those loved ones. These illnesses may be Alzheimer's, other forms of dementia, ALS (amyotrophic lateral sclerosis, or Lou Gehrig's disease), congestive heart failure, metastatic cancer,

COPD (chronic obstructive pulmonary disease), AIDS, Huntington's disease, or other progressive illnesses that eventually can't be controlled. As a loved one's condition changes, so does the role of the caregiver. That was the case with Bea. Had she developed her renal failure fifteen years earlier, caregiving would have been limited to months. But in 2008 the prognosis indicated at least another five years of life. She had a nephew who doted on her and willingly accepted the role of primary caregiver. While the progression of the illness was slow, it resulted in constant changes in the type of caregiving required. When incontinence and poor bowel control became a problem, Bea's modesty and her nephew's discomfort with handling bodily wastes affected their relationship. The favorite aunt developed an array of problems because she was embarrassed to ask her nephew to change her absorbent underpants. The doting nephew began having second thoughts when his idealized image of caregiving was replaced by reality. Because he did not understand how his role would change as the illness progressed, the nephew grew distant from his aunt, and she felt isolated at a time when she most needed compassion.

From the moment of diagnosis, caregivers begin a journey of adjustment. We adjust to the needs of our loved ones. We adjust to our new lives. We adjust to continuous changes in our loved ones' physical and emotional conditions. We adjust to the misunderstanding of friends and strangers about our loved ones' behavior and our own. And finally, we adjust to the loss of our loved ones' personalities or lives. Our roles as caregivers continually evolve, leaving behind expectations of what "should be" as if they were 1970s computers.

Adapt to the Fluctuations

The arc of dying, from the moment of the diagnosis to grieving after a loved one's death, is characterized by a constant flux in emotions.

Change isn't orderly, and at times it is barely understandable. What a loved one felt last week will not necessarily be what she feels today, or tomorrow, or perhaps in the next two hours. That's what happened with a seventy-five-year-old woman I served who had breast cancer. Her husband was devoted to her, and even though he was eighty he assumed the role of primary caregiver to provide for her physical and emotional needs. I would sit next to Betty's bed when Rich did his weekly errands. We would eat chocolate, one of the few foods that she could taste and one that gave her great pleasure. Each week I brought her a chocolate bar from another country, and she would savor a small piece, commenting on the texture and butterfat content.

"I can't believe how much Rich is doing," Betty said to me on our Belgian chocolate day. "He's constantly caring for me. I told him we could afford someone to come in and help, but he insists on doing everything himself. He says it's important to him. God, I'm blessed!"

For three months she would repeat her accolades during my weekly visits as we sampled new European delights. About three weeks before she died, our conversations started changing. She began complaining that Rich would forget to do certain things, that he wasn't as attentive as he had been, and that he wasn't as caring. She even began wondering if he was seeing another woman when he was supposedly doing errands. On one occasion, she reprimanded him in my presence when he was ten minutes late getting back.

Was he changing? Based on three months of interactions, I didn't think so. If anything, I saw a greater attention to her needs. What was changing was Betty's fear of suffocating as her lung capacity decreased. Rich was aware of this, and when Betty berated him, he would apologize, saying, "I'll try to do better, honey." He understood that his wife's condition was changing, and that along with the changes came an uncontrollable fear that he couldn't reduce. Although her anger was directed at him, he knew it wasn't about him. Life was changing for Betty, and therefore it changed for Rich. Had he reacted to her as if her condition hadn't changed, he might have drifted away from her, leading to a more difficult death for her. Instead, he adapted to the changes occurring in his wife's body and mind. During one visit, after Betty had made abusive accusations and we left her room, he turned to me with tears in his eyes and said, "I know how afraid she is. I don't expect her to think about my feelings." Just as happened to Betty, your loved one's emotions will fluctuate. The fluctuations may sometimes result from the pain; at other times they may reflect your loved one's realization of what is happening to him, or his recognition of the lack of time he has left to complete unfinished business, what he is putting you through, or a future he won't have. Regardless of the reason, adapt.

HOW MUCH TRUTH?

Physicians who aren't involved in palliative care (pain reduction) or end-of-life issues are often unsure how to transmit the news of a progressive or terminal illness. This inability may be due to a lack of training or the almost universal view among physicians that death is the enemy. Worse, the deaths of their patients may say to them something about their competency. Accolades are given to those who save lives. Nobody applauds physicians when they can't stop the progression of an illness. So it is understandable that many physicians have difficulty conveying the news of a chronic or terminal prognosis. Unfortunately, their discomfort may affect the explanation of a loved one's status.

Insist on an Accurate Prognosis

When my brother-in-law had just undergone neurosurgery for the removal of a malignant brain tumor, the surgeon came into the waiting room to discuss the outcome with my wife, our two adult children, and me.

"The surgery went very well," he said.

My wife and children looked relieved. I was familiar with the aggressiveness of this type of cancer and wasn't satisfied with "very well." So I asked, "How much of the tumor were you able to remove?"

"Well, I couldn't get all the tentacles; they were too deep in the brain."

"Does that mean they'll grow back?"

He hesitated before answering. "Most likely."

"Are you saying that his condition is terminal?"

I knew this was a conversation that was uncomfortable for everyone. But I had been a bedside hospice volunteer for more than four years by then, and I knew the importance to families of understanding what would be happening to a loved one and how soon it would occur. And I knew that my contact with my brother-in-law's surgeon might be limited to this one meeting.

"Well, yes," the surgeon said, "but he might have at least a few years." I knew this was a confusing message he was giving my family. On the one hand, it was clearly a terminal prognosis, but on the other, it could be years until my brother-in-law died. Emotionally, there is finality in the word *terminal*. Qualifying it by saying, "It could be years," softened and distorted the prognosis.

"Is two years the maximum or average?" I asked.

"It's a wide range."

I thought this was a strange response to a specific question. This was a surgeon who kept up with the literature and had an international reputation for pioneering important surgical techniques. Yet he was equivocating as if he were a first-year intern. I think it became clear to him that I would continue pressing for definitive information.

"With tumors such as my brother-in-law's, what's the survival range?"

"Three months to one and a half years." My wife and children looked shocked. "But we can't be sure until the lab results come back," he quickly added.

"How sure are you of the prognosis, based on your experience?" I asked.

"I don't like giving one without the data."

"But if you had to give it right now, what would it be?"

"Very aggressive."

Not only was he becoming irritated with my questions, but I could also see that my insistence on answers was upsetting my family. Yet there was one last question I had to ask. It was one that I knew could make the difference between my brother-in-law having a more peaceful death and one that might be haunted by regrets.

"Will you, or should we, tell him the prognosis?" I asked.

The surgeon was startled. "I don't think anyone should tell him. I've found that patients live longer when they don't know their terminal status."

I didn't expect this response from him. The idea that truthful prognoses should be withheld from patients is dated. In 1961, only 10 percent of physicians surveyed believed it was correct to tell a patient of a fatal cancer diagnosis. By 1979, 97 percent felt that such disclosures were correct. Yet here was an internationally renowned surgeon in 2006 buying into an antiquated notion of routinely not informing patients about a terminal prognosis. I learned from this and other experiences that the priority of many physicians is to extend the lives of patients, without taking into account the quality of life they leave them with.

Physicians should clearly state, at least to you, that the prognosis is stable, progressive, or terminal. Vagueness can lead to consequences that, although unintentional, are detrimental to caregivers and loved ones. That was the case with my brother-in-law. He refused to believe he was dying because the surgeon never used *terminal* or an equivalent word. The conversations he had with the surgeon over the next six months always contained qualifications. As the tumor regrew, causing paralysis and delusions, the time grew shorter for my brother-in-law to do the things necessary to prepare to die and for my family to prepare to serve him. Yet little planning was possible, because he refused to believe he was dying. His admiration for the surgeon made any attempt to talk about dying futile. According to him, "The surgeon is internationally known. He never said my condition was terminal. How could you and my sister know as much as him?" We eventually asked the surgeon to write a letter clearly describing my brother-in-law's condition. Only after that letter did he begin tying up the loose ends of his life, and then we could make major caregiving preparations.

What to Tell a Loved One?

It's not unusual that caregivers are informed of progressive or terminal prognoses before loved ones are. This is often true when a loved one is elderly and a relative accompanies him to the physician's office, or the physician is not familiar with the patient's cultural or religious values. Out of respect, a physician will often ask family members if their loved one should be told about her status. What would you decide if the decision were left to you? Simple answers such as "She has a right to know" or "What's the point of telling her she'll die soon?" gloss over the complexities of the question.

At the children's hospice where I volunteered, if a child asked if he or she was dying, it was the organization's policy to tell the truth. Everyone, including me, dreaded having the question asked. After all, how do you tell a child that he is dying? But it happened.

"I think I'm dying," a seven-year-old said to me while we were playing Chutes and Ladders.

"Why do you think that?" I asked.

"I'm wearing diapers and my tummy hurts all the time."

"Do you remember when you came here and how much everything hurt?"

"Yes."

"The medicine you're taking now makes the pain go away, doesn't it?"

"Uh-huh."

"That medicine makes your tummy hurt a little and also gives you loose poops."

"Okay. My turn!"

He wasn't asking me if he was dying, but rather wondering why he wasn't able to control his bowels and why his stomach constantly ached. His question was related to the effects of palliative drugs, not existential issues of life and death. I learned that the concept of "death" for a young child is not the same as it is for a sixty-year-old, and the circumstances surrounding the question often mitigate absolutes. There are no easy answers when it comes to conveying a progressive or terminal prognosis to a loved one. Ideas such as "He has a right to know" make theoretical sense when there is no context. Involve a real person with a history that a caregiver is intimately familiar with, and absolutes become equivocal. When the neurosurgeon suggested that nobody tell my brother-in-law he was dying, my wife agreed with him, and, as important as I thought it was to be honest, I acquiesced. She knew her brother far better than I did. What she knew was that honesty following the operation wouldn't be beneficial, and there would be time later to have the important discussion.

For many people, the question of whether to tell may be moot, especially if a physician has been honest, a loved one has asked the physician about the prognosis, or a loved one's body has sent unmistakable messages. But in many cases, caregivers are faced with this very difficult decision. Whether to tell shouldn't be based on caregivers' own comfort or discomfort with the question. Rather, such decisions should involve the expressed wishes of loved ones or, in the absence of previously expressed wishes, their history.

In some situations, it is uncertain if loved ones really want to know they have been given a terminal prognosis. I think those situations are the most difficult. Caregivers then must assume the role of facilitator, reflecting back questions. For example, following a very difficult day, a husband said to his wife, "I'm not sure I'm going to make it this time." Instead of confirming or denying her husband's concerns, she responded by asking a question: "Why do you think that?" There are times when a loved one just needs a nonjudgmental sounding board. If loved ones need to believe they will survive, who are we to tell them it's a futile hope? When a friend of my mother was dying of stomach cancer, all her friends would gather by her bedside and reassure her that she was looking better. A week before her death, she weighed less than ninety pounds and couldn't keep any food or liquids down. Everyone knew she was dying, but they also knew she did not want to face her mortality, and in accordance with what they knew, they obliged her. My wife knew her brother's needs far better than I did, and she was right in not forcing him at that time to realize he was dying.

THE ROLE OF DEATH
IN LIFE AND CAREGIVING

In many Japanese towns and villages, the symbols of death and life intermingle. In a cemetery in one town, I saw small stone statues of children adorned with fresh flowers and covered with brightly colored sweaters, as if this human touch could be transferred to their spirits. On one side of the cemetery stood a tea shop where people leisurely drank tea, and on the other side a clothing store decorated with twinkling neon lights, which sold clothes bearing nonsensical English word combinations to teenagers.

In the West, we place our cemeteries away from our everyday

lives, as if there were an impermeable barrier separating life and death. Living without the willingness to acknowledge death makes living less meaningful. Similarly, we cannot understand sweetness without also knowing bitterness. We delude ourselves by pretending that death — the elephant in the room — will go away if we just ignore it. The Persian poet Rumi wrote a version of the wonderful allegory of the elephant more than eight hundred years ago. And it is as insightful today as when it originally appeared.

In the Middle Ages, death was viewed as a natural, inevitable event. Life then was short, and the possibility of dying was always present. As we became technologically more advanced, death was delayed. Medical devices and miracle drugs — unimaginable to our ancestors — created the illusion that we and our loved ones could live indefinitely. We have always known that this isn't true, but with a little effort the pretense can persist. However, the illusion comes with a price. Death becomes disconnected from life. It remains in the shadows and is spoken about euphemistically. It becomes a sharp point from which we recoil. And when it becomes imminent, we often don't know how to react.

Death Is a Community Event

Death is not a solo event, confined to a single person. Rather, it is shaped by the dynamic interaction between the person who is dying and those who are not, by those who understand there's little time left and, perhaps, by others who falsely believe life can be endless. There is a saying that death is to living as the elephant is to the jungle; both leave the biggest footprint. Yet we in Western society treat death's impending approach as if it had the impact of a squirrel's footprint. We use words such as *eternal sleep*, *going back home*, *passing away*, *crossing over*, and many other phrases that attempt to soften the end of life. As afraid as we may be, our fears become magnified when it comes to being honest with our children. We hide the knowledge that a loved one is dying, believing that our action will spare them emotional distress. And when they pointedly ask about the absence or condition of a relative, we often become as disfluent as if we were answering a young child's question about how babies are made.

When Thomas Merton, the great Catholic theologian, was a child, in the 1920s, and his mother lay dying in a hospital only a few miles from where he was staying with his father's friends, he was never allowed to see her. The belief at the time was that it would be such a traumatic event that it would scar him for life. Their communication was limited to the exchange of letters. As an adult, Merton lamented that the well-intentioned desire to protect him from the reality of death left many open wounds. It's been more than eighty years since that misguided belief prevented a young boy and his mother from saying their final good-byes. Yet today little has changed. Many still look at death as if it were an embarrassing relative they would prefer didn't attend family events. Unfortunately, we perpetuate our own discomfort or fear of death by transferring it to our children, and they to their children.

Bring closer to you the things you fear the most. Whenever you're feeling uncomfortable with a caregiving issue, lean into it rather than running away. Running away perpetuates the fear. Leaning into it makes it more intimate and therefore more understandable and manageable.

Treat Death as an Ongoing Event

Most people perceive death as a single event, analogous to a light switch — the light is on or it's off; someone is alive, then they aren't. But death is a process that spans time, beginning with a terminal prognosis and ending with the recovery of a caregiver's joy. Some would argue that it begins with our first breath. How loved ones deal with it is analogous to a square dance where partners are continuously changing. But instead of other dancers, loved ones' hands may be held by fears, beliefs, an unresolved past, and a nonexistent future. Into this scene step caregivers who want to help their loved ones. They learn that caregiving and death are far more complex than they anticipated.

Imagine standing on a small board that is balanced on a large ball. Your task is to stay upright. With each slight shift of your body, the ball moves and you need to readjust your balance. Now imagine that next to you is another person on a similar device, and the task for each of you is to hold on to the ends of a single stick. Your movements will affect the movements of the other person, and vice versa. Having a progressive illness is like perpetually standing on that balance board. Just when a loved one begins to accept what is happening to him physically or emotionally, the ball moves and the balance he believed was established disappears. It can shift because the illness moves into a new phase or he has second thoughts about granting forgiveness to someone, or the pain he thought was controlled becomes so intense it makes thinking impossible, or his previous acceptance of his imminent or eventual death no longer looks tolerable, or the forgiveness he has been waiting for doesn't come. And all during these adjustments, you are there, still holding on to the end of the stick, both you and your loved one hoping not to pull the other down.

DEFINING THE "GOOD DEATH"

Everyone would like his or her loved one to have a "good death," whether it will occur in months or years. The question of what a "good death" is has been debated throughout history. When people are asked what the phrase means, their explanations are usually based on their values. It's like when you ask people, "What is beauty?" Their answers are as diverse as the people you ask. The son of a woman I served had a very simple definition of a good death: "Ideally, her death will come in her sleep and be quick and painless. She wouldn't know what hit her." While this type of death may be preferable, a significant number of deaths occur after a lingering illness. So, we're still left with the question of what a good death is for people whose end isn't instantaneous. I've served a number of people whose deaths I thought were good, and others whose deaths I felt weren't. Common to most good deaths was a psychological peacefulness that overshadowed physical pain. Two things that contributed to this peacefulness were the compassion expressed through the practical comforts provided by caregivers, and the loved one's ability to tie up life's loose ends.

Provide Practical Comforts

Scholars identify characteristics such as "authenticity," "independence," and "autonomy" as essential for the good death. Some religious leaders maintain that a good death depends on the acceptance of spiritual doctrine. The essayist H.L. Mencken wrote, "We are here and it is now. Further than that all human knowledge is moonshine." Many of us who serve the dying appreciate Mencken's blunt assessment of life and, by extension, death. One of my patients told me that she never thought about "autonomy," but she wondered if her husband was okay with wiping the drool from her chin. Another patient with limited bowel control wasn't concerned about notions of "independence," but he worried how his wife would react to changing an absorbent brief and cleaning his bottom. A Fortune 500 executive who was estranged from his children didn't want to become "authentic"; he wanted his children's forgiveness.

Concepts such as autonomy, self-image, and independence are as relevant to those I have served as an architect's discussion of physics is to a carpenter wanting to choose the right nail to use for hardwood. Both the carpenter and dying loved ones live in a world of practicalities. The carpenter wants to know which nail to use. Loved ones search for a gentle way of exiting life. As life is reduced to the basics because of a chronic or terminal illness, ways of dealing with it become concrete. The "good death" for those I have served involved the fulfillment of needs as diverse as the patients, and were not related to concepts presented by academicians and some religious writers. Trying to fit the reality of dying into a theory or religious doctrine about death is equivalent to attempting to put on a pair of jeans three sizes too small. You can do it, but it's going to be very uncomfortable. This doesn't mean there is no place for religion in caregiving. For some caregivers and loved ones, it is a crucial component. But religious doctrine is often very distant from the daily needs of loved ones.

Tie Up Loose Ends

Even when life is going well, there is a certain satisfaction in knowing that things have been completed, whether this means paying all the bills before going on vacation or completing a list of chores before going back to work on Monday. The need to complete things is even more critical near the end of life. The importance of certain things is obvious, such as giving thanks or asking for forgiveness. But others are symbolic in creating a sense of closure as life ends. In chapter 6, I discuss in greater detail the specific types of loose ends I've found that patients believed they needed to tie up before dying.

FINAL THOUGHTS

When most people write about long-term caring, they focus on those who need care, and they tend to gloss over the enormous changes that occur in the life of the caregiver. As I read some of these books, I wondered whether the authors were ever involved in long-term caregiving, or whether their understanding came from a theoretical perspective of what "should be." There is a balance that must be met, not one where the needs of one person trump the other, but where caregivers and loved ones both benefit.

Most longtime caregivers talk about the situation taking charge of what they were able to do. People who never thought they were capable of being compassionate developed caring aspects of their personalities that they continued to use in other settings. Those who viewed life as either black or white began seeing a multitude of shades when they allowed the needs of loved ones to set the agenda. The space occupied by a person who is chronically ill or dying is not only spiritual but also transforming. It's a state of being that is sometimes not understood by family and friends who have little or no involvement. When I wrote *Lessons for the Living: Stories of Forgiveness, Gratitude, and Courage at the End of Life*, I was thrilled with the reviews until I read one from an academic whose teaching encompassed end-of-life issues. She was skeptical that the experiences I wrote about could possibly have been true. It's never pleasant to have your honesty questioned. Once I got past the accusations, I realized that the stories were questionable to her because either she hadn't had the experience of being with a large number of dying people or hadn't allowed herself to be open with them. Caregiving creates a milieu in which the level of connectiveness is unmatched in any other setting. If you remain open, your experiences will change your life in unimaginably positive ways.

If there is one word that should guide you on your journey, it's *acceptance*. We often look at the behavior of others and think, "I wouldn't do it that way." Or, after watching unskillful behaviors (those behaviors that unintentionally hurt), we may say, "How could he do that?" But the one thing that will be made clear in the next two chapters is that the world of caregivers and the world of those who are chronically or terminally ill are very different. Understanding how they differ can lead you to accept what you might not understand. It can also lead you to accept that many of the choices you will make for your loved one will entail identifying the least painful one among the alternatives, rather than the ideal choice.

If caregiving were a static skill, this could be a step-by-step manual, similar to instructions for putting together a child's toy. Just attach A to B and then to C, and so on, and you will have done what is necessary to be a great caregiver. But it's not like that. Caregiving is similar to cooking. For the past fifteen years, I've been given the assignment of making chili for fifty people for our Super Bowl party. I know in advance the items I'll use, but I never follow a recipe. Instead I taste the concoction as I add each new ingredient. If the flavor isn't what I want it to be, I adjust the quantities. It never tastes the same from year to year, yet I'm always asked to do it again the following year. We can strive to be compassionate caregivers, but we rarely know the exact amount of each ingredient that we need in order to make it work. Yet when we prepare well enough, and pay enough attention to what we are doing, both the chili and the service to loved ones turn out well.

You may have already started your journey, or may be about to start it, or may be preparing for one that will eventually happen. Along the way, you will encounter both joy and sharp points. Preparing for the future may be painful. If you focus on the present and implement the suggestions you glean here from other caregivers' experiences, you'll find that the future will be shaped more by what you do now than by regrets about what was left unsaid or undone.

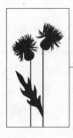

CHAPTER 2

Your World

There's a story about an old man who sees a scorpion clinging to a branch over a fast-moving river. He climbs the tree hoping to save the scorpion before it falls into the water and drowns. He reaches as far as he can, and the scorpion stings him. In agony but undeterred, he tries again, and again the scorpion strikes. A younger man is watching from the shore and sees the scorpion repeatedly sting its potential rescuer. Eventually the younger man says, "Stupid old man! Don't you know that it's in the nature of scorpions to sting?" The old man's hand is swollen to twice its normal size. Writhing in pain, he says, "Yes, just like it's in my nature to save."

Caregiving is a natural condition of being human. We do it for our children and when a loved one or friend becomes ill. Some people choose it as a profession. But continuous caregiving for an extended period of time is not something in our DNA. It involves sacrificing some of our most basic needs for the benefit of others. Done for short periods of time, it can be wonderfully transformative. But when it becomes long-term, the life of a caregiver changes, often in ways that are less than positive. Although some caregivers accept the unwelcome changes as part of the caregiving package, those changes aren't inevitable. The way in which one approaches caregiving will determine the magnitude and impact of both positive and negative changes.

Being a primary caregiver for a loved one with a chronic or terminal illness is analogous to being tossed into a riptide, where you have no control over the general direction of the water, but where you can survive by understanding how the water moves. Fighting the outgoing flow just takes you farther out to sea. Giving up will surely result in drowning. But swimming across the current, modifying what you would normally do in a calm ocean, can allow for escape from the outgoing tide and a return back to shore. Adapting to the situation will do the same for caregivers.

How we approach caregiving reflects our history and our present values. Caregiving, with its immediate consequences, tests one's beliefs. It's one thing to talk about servicing the need of another, and quite another thing to care for someone with, for an example, an infectious disease. There is nothing theoretical about caring for someone, nor a better test of compassion than being the focus of irrational anger. Often the notion of caregiving is associated with self-sacrifice. Although that does occur in caregiving, placing the needs of others over one's own make for a very complicated world for the person who is doing the caring.

CELEBRATE LIFE

We tend to dwell on a loved one's illness as if it constituted the majority of her existence. Doing so allows the rest of a fruitful life to be ignored. It's as if we have given permission to this horrible thing to block out a lifetime of wonderful events. Eventually our loved one's room may become filled with medical supplies and various contraptions that shout out, "Hey, you're sick," or, even more ominously, "You're dying!" That all may be true, but those weeks, months, or few years constitute only a small portion of your loved one's life. Yes, do what needs to be done for someone with a chronic or terminal illness, but don't neglect the wonderful memories of her life with you and the people whose lives she touched. Do it constantly, from the time of her diagnosis to the end of her life.

Talk about Wonderful Past Memories

I would sit for long periods with Jim in his kitchen when Lisa slept. He was a large man who had laid bricks his entire life until he retired, five years before Lisa received a terminal prognosis of congestive heart failure. Unlike her husband, Lisa was very small, and, in the words of Jim, "The disease shrank her to the size of a tiny bird." Jim said the following to me one day.

Neither of us is into the touchy-feely stuff. Lisa and I have been married for almost fifty years. Before we knew she was dying, I don't remember the last time I told her that I loved her. But she knew it by the things I did. We came home from the doctor's office that day, the day Dr. Louis said she would be the one to leave first, and we sat at this kitchen table and had coffee. Mind you, there was nothing special about us sitting here. We did that almost every day. It was a kind of ritual. We never talked when we drank our coffee. She usually had a book, some woman's novel I'd never look at, and I had a newspaper folded back to the sports section, which she wouldn't read even if nothing else was around. We'd sit there every morning, year in, year out, not even looking at each other, just reading and drinking coffee. Well, it usually took us about fifteen minutes to drink a cup. We'd hang around it, you know. Not really drinking it, just being together without fussing.

We started doing the same thing that day when we returned from the doctor's office. I was hiding behind the newspaper when Lisa reached her hand over the table and held mine. I put my paper down and she saw my tears.

"Jim," she said, "I love you. I always have, and I'm sorry I'll be leaving you." Well, I started bawling. Can you imagine that? Me, a guy who never cried. My father taught me that men should hold in their feelings. We must have held each other's hand, not saying anything, for a good five minutes. That was longer than I could ever remember doing that. Finally, I told her how much I loved her and what she had meant to me all these years. It was as if one of my brick walls tumbled over and I was able to say things I hadn't even thought about for years, maybe never..

From that day on, I've told her how important she's been to me. I know I'll miss her when she's gone, but I'll have the memories of the last six months we had together.

Lisa died three weeks later with Jim holding her in his arms. Just as he predicted, he was lonely without her, but at the memorial service he spoke about their last months together and how important it was to him that he was able to relive their wonderful life together by recalling his memories. The grief was still palpable but, I believe, less painful than it would have been had they not had those incredibly honest discussions about their intertwined lives. Instead of being hobbled by what wasn't said and done, he was able to reflect on some of the most honest and meaningful conversations he and his wife ever had.

Giving lesser importance to illness than life is neither a denial of death nor a rejection of reality. Rather, it's a positive view of the role of illness and death in someone's life — both are just the inevitabilities of living. And because they are inevitable, you can treat them with the same importance that you give other things in your loved one's life, such as the love she shared with you, the incredible events she participated in, the good she has done, and everything else that constituted a full life. It's never too early to start these conversations with a loved one. Explore the wonderful things in your loved one's past — not merely in a descriptive way but by talking about what each meant to you.

Remove as Many Medical Items as Possible

The person who has a chronic or terminal illness lives every minute with it. It's there with every discomfort, every movement, and every request for assistance. As the illness progresses, the room he spends most of his time in becomes filled with medical supplies and equipment that only reinforce the dreadfulness of his condition. This may seem like something minor, but removing as many of the items related to the illness as possible can have positive effects. A popular saying among vegetarians is: "You are what you eat." In caregiving, this can be transformed into: "You become what you see."

I was serving a man in his home, where his wife was the primary caregiver. His room was cluttered with the items he most often requested during the day: medicines, diapers, chocks, clean towels, a suction device, an oxygen concentrator, which happened to be loud, and boxes of tissues, which were stacked high. For two months he had been unable to leave his bed other than to sit on the commode. Within his range of vision were things that reinforced the dire circumstances of his condition. These spoke to him of what he had lost and the debilitation that would follow him to his death. Although it was an inconvenience to his wife, I convinced her to move most of the medical items just outside of his room, and to relocate the oxygen concentrator, with its relentless thumping, to a distant room, since the oxygen tube was long enough to snake through the apartment. With those materials moved, we filled the space with items that reflected his past glorious life. Looking at a national award given to him for outstanding sales, for example, had a much more soothing effect than looking at a stack of diapers and a commode.

THOSE UNSPEAKABLE FEELINGS

Someone who has never been a caregiver probably has no idea of the emotional and physical toll it can take. An "outsider" may look at the person providing care and see only unquestioning love and sacrifice. But caregivers silently struggle with the less-than-positive emotions that are intertwined with the genuine love they feel for the people they're caring for. Although caregiving is a complex psychological phenomenon, it's often depicted in the media in one of two ways. One image is that of the adult child who abuses an elderly parent, and the other is the wife who selflessly cares for her husband for twenty years without complaining. Neither of these extremes represents most caregiving situations.

Don't Feel Guilty

I'd been a bedside volunteer for more than five years, sitting with dying patients and their families once or twice a week for up to four continuous hours. Sometimes I'd stayed overnight with patients when I was asked to do a vigil (when a patient was close to death). Regardless of how demanding my responsibilities were, I knew that, when I left the bedside, I'd have three to six days to "recover." It was a time to prepare myself for the next week's activities, which might range from cooking a meal to witnessing a friend's active dying. Downtime — something that allowed me to recharge my batteries — is a luxury many caregivers don't have.

My understanding of what caregivers go through broadened when I was volunteering at the George Mark Children's House, the first freestanding children's hospice in the United States. Besides serving children who are dying, it functions as a facility for respite care. Parents, who may not have had a break from caregiving for years, can drop off a child with a life-threatening illness and take a short vacation, knowing that their child will be competently and compassionately cared for. Listening to parents express how important respite care was for their sanity took me one step closer to understanding the plight of caregivers. That understanding jumped another level when my wife suffered a stroke from a heart arrhythmia and, overnight, my daughter and I became 24/7 caregivers. Fortunately, my wife recovered without any lasting disabilities. But the three-month experience left me with a new and deeper understanding of caregivers' emotions.

One year before my wife's stroke, I had registered for a four-day flute workshop, which, as it turned out, was to take place during her convalescence. It was something I had been dreaming about doing for years. Since I thought my daughter and son would be able to meet all of my wife's physical needs while I was gone, I casually mentioned the workshop to her. I hoped that she would say, "Of course, Stan, go to the workshop, I'll be fine." But the fear on her face made me immediately realize what a bad idea it was. I quickly said, "But I have no intention of going." Although I knew it was necessary to subvert my needs to hers, I couldn't help feeling some resentment — an emotion I was ashamed of having, since I did (and still do) love her. I knew my needs were trivial compared with hers.

In conversation, I've found similar feelings expressed by other people who have been long-term caregivers. Although there is a natural desire to satisfy our own needs, we rarely feel comfortable talking about them. Why? Because the mantle of Mother Teresa is often imposed on us by others or ourselves. Expectations, regardless of the source, can become straitjackets from which even Houdini couldn't have escaped. And for each positive emotion, there is a flip side: with love may come hate, with acceptance comes criticism, and gratitude is sometimes followed by rejection, to name just a few emotions that might occur in a single day. Some caregivers would say within a single hour.

Try to imagine what you might feel after giving up your life to care for an aging parent you dearly love, who screams at you that you aren't doing enough for her because a meal is ten minutes late. And you know that the ingratitude will continue to be expressed until her Alzheimer's changes this unintentionally hurtful behavior into silence. Feeling contradictory emotions is neither right nor wrong. They emerge from situations where the needs of people are in conflict. During times when you wonder if your needs will ever be met, don't push away the feeling. Caring for a loved one is emotionally and physically draining, and you will feel many contradictory emotions. Be kinder to yourself than you may think you deserve.

Resent the Illness and Not the Loved One

It's difficult to accept a loved one's use of painful words to describe your level of caring. You know what you've sacrificed, and that what you have given is exemplary. And you know that illness, either stable or progressive, shapes almost everything your loved one experiences. The constant presence of something that is life-altering creates a perceptual lens that can distort what is being seen or heard. Unfortunately, caregivers often bear the brunt of their loved ones' responses to the distortions. Intellectually, you know this, but it still hurts. A woman with ovarian cancer was constantly affected by the uncertainty of when her pain would subside and how long the relief would last. Her husband would take her outside for a stroll in her wheelchair, and instead of thanking him, she would fuss whenever he allowed her chair to hit a crack in the sidewalk. He would fix her favorite dessert, and instead of being grateful, she would quiz him on the ingredients, fearing that one would exacerbate the pain. Fortunately, he understood that it was the disease that was criticizing him. "It's okay," he said to me. "I understand that we live in different worlds. That's not Marge who's being cruel, it's the cancer."

Another caregiver, whose husband had ALS, felt she wasn't successful at finding an antidote to her husband's cruel words. "I hate what this disease has done to me and my family. It's taken away my future and my son's. After caring for Bill for twelve straight hours, I have a hard time listening to his criticism. I still love him dearly, and I know he's talking through his disease. It gets hard for me to turn the other cheek, but I do it, again and again." We talked about her belief that there was nothing she could do other than accept her husband's unskillful words and the pain that they caused her. I felt there was another approach — defusing them. It's the guiding principle of Aikido, a martial art that teaches you how to defend yourself while protecting your attacker. Instead of allowing your attacker to hit you, you gently turn him away, dissipating the blow's power. Defending yourself from a loved one involves understanding that the invectives thrown at you reflect his attempts to deal with an untenable situation, not something you did wrong. Protecting your loved one from you requires the type of restraint used when a drunk who can barely stand picks a fight. Gracefully accept those criticisms you know have no merit, apologize, and try to move on.

But there are times when, as much as we want to, we can't. A father with dementia said to his daughter who had cared for him for years, "You're such a klutz!" when she dropped a plate. "You've never done anything right in your life!" Was it thoughtless? Probably. But was it hurtful? Only if his daughter believed it was true. But what if she looked at the intention of the words, rather than their effects? If she accepted that he was consumed with fragmented thoughts and didn't even realize this was his daughter, how is it possible to be hurt by his words? If caregivers are to avoid taking things personally, they need to look beyond seemingly hurtful actions and examine the intention. Why would a father whose daughter has given up her life to care for him be vindictive? Most likely he wouldn't be. His anger and ingratitude say more about the chaos he was experiencing than anything else. You will learn much from your loved one, some of which will come from the absence of what you desire. Take each treasure into your heart. There will be much wisdom in it.

It's All Right to Wish It Were Over

With my wife, there was never an issue of her not surviving. But many caregivers realize that, no matter what they do, a loved one will not live despite months or years of compassionate and competent care. At times the futility of a caregiver's efforts becomes a dominant feature of her thinking. And that's when the guilt-ridden thought "I wish it were over; I hope he dies soon" may pop up.

Hoping for the death of a loved one is not only difficult to talk about but also troublesome to contemplate. It becomes easier when the motivation is related to the discomfort experienced by your loved one or a dramatic decline in the quality of his life. A couple who had lived together for more than fifty years were devoted to each other. As the wife's ability to breathe became more impaired because of emphysema, the quality of her life dramatically declined. Every day her husband prayed that her life would end. Not because of his caregiving responsibilities — he viewed them as a gift — but because of the pain she was enduring. But often the wish reflects the consuming nature of caregiving. I knew that the changes I needed to make in my lifestyle to care for my wife would end shortly. But with many chronic illnesses, such as various forms of dementia, it may be years until a loved one dies. And as the disease progresses, the demands on the caregiver increase.

A husband who was an executive at a leading company in San Francisco resigned when his wife was diagnosed with a slowly advancing but terminal illness. Although he could have hired someone to care for his wife, he wanted to do it himself. After three months, he recognized that the reality of being a full-time caregiver overshadowed the angelic vision of what he thought it would be like. He still loved her and knew he had made the right decision to resign, but he missed the position he had sacrificed. He told me that, late in the evening after caring for his wife the entire day and preparing her for bed, he would sit at the kitchen table and relax for the first time.

With a glass of bourbon in hand and his wife finally asleep and without pain, he wished it were over for both his wife and his caregiving responsibilities.

I have known caregivers who pushed away the sharp point of wishing everything were over, and those who brought the unthinkable closer. Trying to pretend the feeling doesn't exist won't make it go away. But acknowledging that your life has changed, often in ways that are not repairable, can lead to an acceptance of your situation. And that moment of acceptance can be transformative in caregiving. I once asked a hospice nurse how she was able to let go of patients. "If I'd believed I could save any of the more than four thousand patients I've served," she told me, "I would have stopped doing this years ago. I know I'll lose every one. What allows me to continue is knowing that, when I leave the bedside, I have done whatever was possible to make that moment as good as it could be for that patient. I don't save anyone, but I do add to their comfort."

I believe others' experiences of long-term caregiving, in the cases of both chronic and terminal illness, are in many ways similar to what the hospice nurse expressed. If you focus on what you can do *at the moment* to ease your loved one's discomfort, many things fall into place. Changing a pair of absorbent briefs is no longer a distasteful chore, it's a way to help a loved one to regain the dignity of not lying in a soiled garment. Redoing a meal is not giving in to an unreasonable demand, it's removing one more irritant a loved one is experiencing as a result of the cruelty of the illness. Accepting the unrealistic directions of an elderly demented parent is not a futile gesture, but rather an effort that may help her hold on to a world that is disintegrating.

Don't Blame Anyone

Finding someone to blame for a chronic or terminal prognosis is natural, but it's a reaction that rarely leads to anything positive. You may find yourself thinking one of the following.

- If only she had exercised more.
- If only he had quit smoking earlier.
- If only he had eaten a little less junk food.

"If only" statements do immense damage even if they are based on compelling facts. They not only contribute to a loved one's guilt if spoken aloud, but they also often reflect unproven ideas. A friend of mine who ran marathons and ate only organic foods died of a heart attack at fifty. He ran every day, not because he enjoyed running, but because he believed it would increase his lifespan. Unbeknown to him, his defective heart valve was always on the verge of failing. A relative who had been smoking two packs a day since he was sixteen, and whose idea of exercise was retrieving the morning paper from his front stoop, is now in his eighties and is confounding everyone because he's still alive.

There are times when it may be possible to assign blame, especially in very clear-cut cases. Say, for example, a doctor examines a loved one and says, "If you don't bring your weight down, you'll develop diabetes, and that could lead to a heart attack or stroke because of your increased blood pressure and arterial sclerosis." Your loved one doesn't listen and, just as predicted, diabetes develops, followed by a severe heart attack. He becomes debilitated and you become his long-term caregiver. Even though you love him, you're filled with anger. How could he have done that to himself — and you? Why didn't he just listen to the doctor? Why didn't he change his lifestyle? Looking back at "if only" scenarios does little other than to place you in a time frame that can't be changed. The Buddhist nun and teacher Pema Chödrön explained it most eloquently, saying that looking to the past is like sitting backward on a train. You can see where you have been, but not where you are going. Blame in the form of accusations may allow you to feel a sense of justice, but it won't provide guidance for what to do in the present or the future. The next time you're inclined to think about an "if only" scenario, ask yourself if there is anything in your just accusation that can help you or your loved one now or in the future.

You're Doing the Best You Can

Years ago, when my life was in turmoil, I decided to spend a weekend at the Shasta Abbey Buddhist Monastery in Northern California. When the abbot asked if anyone wished to receive counseling, I raised my hand. The next day I entered a room and saw a monk who was in his twenties — less than half my age at that time. My reluctance to share my life's problems with him faded after a few minutes, and I forgot that he probably had no experience with marriage or children. I spoke freely about the various unskillful things I had done as a father and husband. After about twenty minutes I stopped and he remained silent. Slowly he said, "Stan, we do the best we can, given the circumstances of our lives." Then he rose and left the room. It took me a while to understand the importance of his words. We rarely act in a vacuum. What we do and say are often products of what precedes our actions, including the events swirling around us.

I've spoken with numerous caregivers who've chastised themselves for "not doing a better job." One caregiver related to me her feelings about having had to decide whether to allow her father to die. His physicians had declared him brain-dead, and he was unable to survive without artificial means. For one day she wrestled with a decision, eventually allowing the removal of the medical devices that sustained him. Two years after his death, she still wondered if she had done the right thing, or whether she should have preserved his life for a few more days or weeks, hoping there would be some sign of brain activity.

Often guilt can come from less dramatic events. I recently helped a caregiver find triggers that might be causing her husband's agitated behavior. She had done a marvelous job, finding several, but she felt frustrated at not finding all of them. "I need to get everything right," she insisted. Instead of realizing what a wonderful gift she'd given her husband, who had Alzheimer's, she couldn't get past the few mistakes she made. We do the best we can within a world whose demands often outpace our capabilities.

THE DAY-TO-DAY WORK OF CAREGIVING

Long-term caregiving is a mixture of exhaustion, never-ending routines, moments of indescribable compassion, episodes of depression, spiritual fulfillment, and, with some loved ones, painfully witnessing the dreadful progression of the illness. Understanding how to deal with each factor may help minimize the negative factors and maximize the positive ones.

Expect Exhaustion

As a caregiver, even when you are relaxing, you are still doing something. You may be observing, worrying, and often waiting for something to happen. "Since I started taking care of Louis three months ago," a caretaker said, "I've been exhausted. I have help come in for two hours a day so I can just lie down on my bed and catch some sleep. But no matter how quiet it is, as soon as I hear anything from his room, I wonder what's happening to him." Assume that, if not now, then eventually you will need respite care in order to take a walk, sleep in an adjoining room, or do anything else that produces emotional or physical rest.

We often want to give as much as we physically and emotionally can to our loved ones, and in doing so we may take ourselves beyond our capacity to function well. Unfortunately, the closer we come to exceeding that capacity, the more likely it is that we will reduce our ability to give. We can take a tip from professional baseball coaches. Pitching coaches keep statistics on the maximum number of pitches a pitcher can throw before he begins to give up too many hits. The coach rarely waits until that number arrives before taking a pitcher out of the game. But there is no coach to make the decision for you when it's time to come out of the game. Ask for respite care not when you have reached your limit but well before that point. Caregiving is not a solo endeavor. You will need help, and asking for it doesn't mean you've stopped caring for your loved one. In fact, seeking help is an expression of love for the person you are caring for. The more exhausted you become, the less effective and attentive you'll be.

Accept Change as Inevitable

Just as the life of your loved one is changing, so is yours. Both of you are coming to terms with a world characterized by sinkholes. Parts of her life and yours — parts that were separate or connected — are disappearing. With this change, your identities may change and certain needs may go unfulfilled. One caregiver said, "Every day is different. I thought I understood the importance of not being attached to things that were changing. But when my husband developed Alzheimer's, it wasn't just a matter of letting go of the person he had been before the illness; it was letting go, almost every day, of the person he had developed into the previous day."

Change is difficult for everyone. Just when you think you have adjusted to the caregiving requirements of the illness, it progresses, and once again you go through the process of accepting the changes in your loved one's physical requirements and adjusting to who she is becoming. Even when we know loved ones have changed because of a chronic or terminal illness, we often expect them to react to events as if everything were the same. You wonder how your loved one could be so inconsiderate, knowing what you have given up. She wonders where your compassion went when she needed it the most. Both of you are living in different worlds with some connections between them. Neither deliberately tries to hurt the other, yet both get hurt. So what do you do? For starters, explain to your loved one that sometimes you're not as sensitive as you'd like to be, and ask for her help in providing you with feedback so you can change. You can also explain that you may not understand what she is experiencing unless she shares those feelings with you.

Observe before Judging

As a communicative disorders therapist and a professor, I taught my students the importance of observing. It's something we often ignore before drawing conclusions about why a person says or does something different or unexpected. Edmund Husserl, an early-twentieth-century philosopher, believed that not only in science but also in social relationships, judging before observing distorts what we see. The same is true for the words and actions of loved ones who are chronically or terminally ill. Just observing, without making any initial judgments, may result in understanding why a person says or does something in particular. One of my hospice patients was perpetually angry with everyone, including me. He was dying of hepatitis and was always bitter about everything. His outbursts caused many people to avoid interacting with him. Instead of walking away during a series of rants at staff members, I remained in the background, watching and listening. What I noticed was that his anger was usually triggered when he was told something would happen but wasn't asked for his input: Breakfast will be ready at eight. The massage therapist will be here at four. Your next dose of medicine will be at one o'clock.

"John," I said, "Would you like me to bring up your laundry now or later?"

There was nothing skillful about my statement. What I did differently was to give him a choice. Giving him the dignity of being in control of one simple thing resulted in greater acceptance of me as a caregiver. If I had rushed to a judgment that this was a man angry about dying, I would have reacted differently to him. But by observing first, I realized that his anger was related to the belief that he wasn't being treated as a cognitively intact human being — something he was until his death. Take your time in observing what occurs when loved ones do or say something unexpected or out of character. What immediately preceded it? What were you doing? What was simultaneously occurring physically and emotionally?

Imagine

In John Lennon's wonderful song "Imagine," he writes about what the world would be like if certain things were different — if there were no countries, we would have peace; if people were fed, there would be no hunger; and if everyone were loving, there would be no anger. Forty years after it was written, it still issues a message that could make the world a far better place than it is. But as a philosophy of caregiving, it can be downright dangerous.

There are many things we don't want to see in our loved ones and ourselves, changes that are frightening and uncomfortable. We hope for things we know won't happen, and we pray for outcomes that, deep within us, we know can never happen. The more we imagine the impossibilities, the less we will be prepared for the realities. I think that in caregiving we always walk a fine line between realistic expectations and hoping the worst won't happen. My brother-in-law always favored the "Imagine" side. As his illness progressed, he became less and less prepared for the reality side. Remain positive, not necessarily about your loved one's recovery or extension of life, but about your ability to provide him or her with a meaningful and loving existence for as long as possible.

Explain to Noncaregivers What They Can't Understand

Uninvolved family members and even professional staff often misunderstand the effects of long-term caregiving. Anna had been caring for her sister Jean for six months. She had given up a job she loved, moved into her sister's one-bedroom apartment, and slept on a couch in the living room. When, as a hospice volunteer, I first met her, she told me of an ongoing conflict she was having with the hospice nurse. The nurse was recommending the use of a morphine derivative to relieve Jean's intense pain from her breast cancer. Anna explained to him that Jean refused to take any narcotics because of the dreadful side effects they had produced in the past. The nurse viewed Anna's unwillingness to even talk to her sister about trying the medication as a dispute between Anna and him. What the nurse didn't realize was that, during the six months of providing compassionate care for Jean, Anna had unsuccessfully tried, to the point of tears, to convince her sister to use this narcotic when it was needed. What Anna expressed to the nurse wasn't hostility but the frustration of not being able to reduce her sister's suffering. Just as the world of the caregiver differs from that of the loved one, so does the caregiver's life differ from the lives of members of the non-intensive-caregiving community. Explain in detail what they don't understand. Being misunderstood by people who have never done long-term caregiving should be expected. You'll have many opportunities to teach them.

Limit Multitasking

We live in an age where multitasking is considered a good thing. With so much to do and so little time to do it, people believe they can do multiple things simultaneously and do all of them effectively. Research has shown that's not the case. We have only a certain amount of concentrative ability. Once you start dividing up your concentration among various activities, the amount you have for each decreases. While this finding makes sense, for many caregivers there isn't an option, other than leaving some tasks undone. That was the case with George, a caregiver who had little help from friends or relatives. His wife was immobile, and he needed to do everything for her. Some activities required his full concentration, such as transferring her from the bed to her wheelchair. During a transfer, he didn't think about anything else, since her bones were brittle and a fall would be disastrous. Intense focus was also important when he painfully explained to her that the illness would continually rob her of the ability to move.

Multitasking during a transfer could have risked his wife's safety. Multitasking while explaining how his wife's body would fail her could have led her to assume George was insensitive. While neither of these two activities should be multitasked, there are many things that can be. For example, when George cooked breakfast, the oatmeal, he knew, required five minutes to cook, the perfect amount of time to empty the dishwasher. When listening to voice messages on the phone, he tidied up the living room. As activities pile up, decide which ones can be multitasked and which require your full attention.

A Caregiver's Bracelet

It's common to have a medical bracelet made for a loved one. It allows emergency personnel to be aware of your loved one's condition and others to know where he lives. But rarely do caregivers think about having their own bracelets made. Unless you never leave the side of your loved one, you too should wear a medical bracelet that indicates the address where your loved one lives, what the problem is, the name of the medical contact person, and his or her phone number. There may be times when you must leave your loved one alone. If anything were to happen to you when you were out of the home, and you weren't able to communicate his location and needs, his safety might be at risk. Some services will keep all the information at a central location, where emergency personnel can access a database.

WHERE TO GET HELP

When you hear a diagnosis that is life-changing for you and your loved one, you may experience a sense of isolation, even if you have concerned family and friends, belong to a supportive spiritual organization, and have been told by professionals that they will be there for you. Some caregivers have described it as feeling as if they were in a pool of quicksand that gradually pulls them under. But you're not alone. There are many sources that can provide help. Some may be familiar, while others may not. The following list discusses some of the most useful sources of emotional, medical, and financial help.

Deal with the Medical Community

You'll need to become familiar with the many physical aspects of a chronic or terminal diagnosis. But both you and your loved one will probably be in shock when you learn of the prognosis, and that's not the easiest time to frame questions or understand answers. Moreover, the likelihood is slim that your loved one's physician will at that time accurately describe the progression of the illness, with all of its difficult and painful stages. Unfortunately, sometimes that never occurs, as was the case with my ALS hospice patient. When I first met her, she was already having difficulty speaking, along with arm and leg weakness. She said she didn't understand what was happening to her. I asked if anyone had explained the progression of her illness. She said nobody had, that they had spoken only about muscular weakness. Although I knew how ALS progressed, I felt uncomfortable explaining it, because I didn't know why she hadn't been told, or, if she had been told, why she was denying it. Instead of answering and possibly giving her information her family didn't want her to have, I contacted the hospice administration. They learned that the family was conflicted about whether to tell their mother the full extent of her prognosis. The issue, which could have been defused early in the disease progression, became a crisis point in the woman's care when her physical condition was rapidly deteriorating and neither family members nor her physician had been truthful with her.

You need to know what to expect as the health of a loved one declines and, when necessary, be ready to explain it in a compassionate and truthful way. With the vast amount of inaccuracies on the Internet, it's better for you to explain it, or to have your doctor explain it, than to let your loved one read about it on an unmonitored website. A good example of how this can be handled is a caregiver whose husband was diagnosed with COPD (chronic obstructive pulmonary disease). She had never been involved in any of the couple's finances. He had run his own successful business and taken care of the couple's personal finances. At the time of the diagnosis, the woman had not paid a household bill in thirty years of marriage, and there was no one who could manage her husband's business when he no longer was able. It was vital for her to know how much time she had before she would need to become responsible for all financial matters. Fortunately, her husband's physician was both competent and compassionate and included the family in every illness-management decision.

But according to many caregivers, there is a great divide in medicine: some medical personnel treat the illness of a person mainly as if it were a puzzle to be solved and seemingly prefer (like Dr. Gregory House on TV) not to talk to their patients; and then there are those whose innate compassion comes out in every interaction. Unfortunately, there is a widely held opinion that, other than in palliative care or hospice, a preponderance of Gregory Houses exists in the medical profession. Ask any physician how much training he or she has had in how to talk with patients or how to tell someone they have a terminal prognosis, and you'll probably find the training is measured in hours. Ideally, you'll find a balance between problem solving and compassion in your physician.

Years ago, I wrote an article on what I called the "white coat syndrome." It's the perception of patients and families that those with white coats hold all the answers. With the proliferation of support groups and information sites on the Internet, the once unassailable position of medical personnel is constantly being questioned. Many in the medical community welcome the collaboration of patients and families, while others dismiss efforts of caregivers to become active participants in the management of an illness. Hold on to a physician of the former type, and contact a support organization for suggestions for replacing the latter.

When my wife had a stroke because of atrial fibrillation, we were at a renowned medical center for stroke and cardiology. I was astonished that the two departments responsible for treating her — neurology and cardiology — offered different suggestions for her treatment when she was discharged. Much to the annoyance of the discharge nurse, I refused to have her released until a senior staff person from neurology and one from cardiology came to the room together and agreed on what we should be doing medically. Fortunately, my wife recovered completely. There may be times when the only thing that stands between adequate and inappropriate care for your loved one is your advocacy. It seems that when specialization is something everybody lauds, especially the medical community, care of the person with an illness or injury may become secondary to solving a puzzle.

Use Senior Centers

Almost every community has a senior center. Some are affiliated with national organizations, while others are local. The range of services they provide varies greatly. Obviously, for someone confined to a bed, senior center services may not be appropriate. Some senior centers have programs for those with specific illnesses, such as dementia. And others will pick up individuals in the morning and bring them home later in the day. The amount of time offered for day care varies greatly.

Some loved ones may be reluctant to go to senior centers. They may not want to leave the house or may fear trying something new. You'll likely find that, as your loved one's illness advances and he becomes more dependent on you, he will display increasing reluctance to separate from you. One strategy is to start using a senior center while your loved one is feeling more independent. Another strategy to make the transition easier is to go with him on the first day, or even on subsequent days, and stay until he feels comfortable. And a third strategy is to have him take something along from home that has produced a sense of familiarity or calmness in the past, such as a favorite hat or shirt, or maybe a picture of you. What you want to help him avoid is the feeling that he is going from a safe, stable environment to one where the structure is unknown.

You'll also need to assume that, just as your loved one's illness is progressing, so are the illnesses of other clients at the senior center, and the stability your loved one encountered yesterday at the center may have changed. As the condition of the other seniors changes, they may no longer be physically able to spend time at the center.

Contact Illness-Related Support Centers

While my patient whose husband had COPD was able to get accurate information about her husband's prognosis, other people I've served weren't so fortunate. If you can't get the information you need to care for your loved one and answer her questions, contact a support organization, such as the American Cancer Society, the Alzheimer's Foundation of America, the Chronic Obstructive Pulmonary Disease Foundation, and so on. You'll find an extensive list in appendix 1; only national and international organizations are listed, since most will refer you to local chapters. As you browse the Internet, you'll find websites devoted only to supplying information; others supply only support; and still others combine both. Sites that are unmonitored or unaffiliated with recognized national organizations might provide inaccurate medical or treatment information. Some sites offer wonderful emotional support, while others may discuss intervention protocols that are unproven and sometimes harmful. At one time during my brother-in-law's disease progression, he began contacting people whose websites promised miraculous cures. What he received was expensive interventions that didn't stop the disease's progression. As one of his caregivers, I needed to balance his need to believe the cancer was curable with the predatory practices of unscrupulous quacks. When he eventually accepted that his condition was terminal, it was no longer necessary for me to monitor his contacts.

Many illness-based associations have valuable and no-cost programs to help you once a loved one has been diagnosed with an illness. Some organizations may send a care consultant to your house to meet with you and your family to discuss the illness and answer questions. Others with limited staffing may require a visit to their clinic or office. Staff can develop an individualized plan and help you navigate the maze of available services. Some organizations can assess the prescriptions your loved one is taking and act as your advocate while working with your doctor.

Use Advocates to Navigate Governmental Agencies

Many caregivers have little choice other than to give up their jobs to care for a loved one. Savings become exhausted, assets are sold, and few acceptable financial choices remain to them. Many people are then forced to choose between paying for food and medicine and paying everyday living expenses. "Forced into bankruptcy" is a phrase commonly used to describe long-term caregivers. Help is available, but often the maze placed in front of caregivers is formidable. You can try navigating the resources of available governmental assistance listed in appendix 3 on your own, but I advise you to do it with an advocate. The paperwork can seem unending, the regulations confusing, and the bureaucracy more concerned with meeting all legal requirements than with displaying compassion. Start with a local support organization for your loved one's illness. Your advocate will have up-to-date information and will help you fill out the appropriate forms, will make phone calls to agencies, and may even accompany you to the agencies' offices.

Use Paratransit Services

Many local agencies have vans available to transport individuals with disabilities. Some local agencies provide taxi scrip that you can use to purchase rides with any private transportation company. This can be used for required medical visits or just to take your loved one to visit a friend or a favorite place. Reservations are usually required at least a few days in advance. You'll be told approximately when the paratransit van will arrive and when it will pick up your loved one and you to return to your home. When I was serving a hospice patient who had prostate cancer, we would take a paratransit van from his house to a barbershop in San Francisco's Chinatown during my visits. With little hair left, he had no need for a weekly haircut. However, it was an opportunity for him to meet with old friends. They all knew about his standing appointment and would arrange their schedules to be there, whether or not they needed a haircut. Many people think about the use of a paratransit service only for necessary trips to a physician's office or to governmental agencies to complete forms. But it can provide you and your loved one with an opportunity to escape the confines of your home.

Use Meals On Wheels

Sometimes the last thing you want to do after hours of nonstop caregiving is cook a meal. Instead of microwaving an unappetizing package of processed food, contact your local Meals On Wheels chapter.

The Meals On Wheels Association of America is the oldest and largest national organization representing local and community-based senior nutrition programs. More than five thousand local chapters can be found, in all fifty states and in the U.S. territories. These programs provide more than one million daily meals to seniors who need them. Some programs serve meals at congregate locations like senior centers, some programs deliver meals directly to the homes of seniors whose mobility is limited, and many programs provide both services. There are also local organizations that provide the same services. Most are free or require a small donation.

Join Social Networks

Internet social networks are profuse and serve many functions. For example, in Yahoo! Groups, searching for the term *caregivers* yields 2,966 groups with *caregiver* in the title or description. Adding *loved one* to the search reduces it to 228. Making it even more specific (for example, by searching for *caregiver Alzheimer's*) shrinks it to a manageable number. Such networks can be used as contact with the outside world when caregiving is constant and you need a safe place to vent your frustration. On these sites, caregivers can also be reassured by other caregivers that what they are feeling or experiencing is normal. And such groups can provide helpful information. Although very few sites are set up to do just one thing, the focus of the group is often clear. Some are more factual and provide valuable information about the illness, while others act as an escape valve for frustrations. Some are "open" groups allowing anyone to join. Others require approval by a group moderator. An extensive list appears in appendix 2.

Problems can crop up on such sites, however. A caregiver may go to a site desperately looking for advice, and in response to his question other members may share similar problems without providing answers. On one site, a woman expressed her despondency over the death of her husband and asked what she could do to help herself get out of bed each day. The other members of the group were very supportive and told her about their own experiences, but they provided no suggestions for getting on with her life. When I looked at three months' worth of archived posts on that site, I saw that over time her comments had become increasing more desperate. She kept asking for advice, and she received support but no answers. Her last post alarmed everyone in the group. She felt that, since no one could provide her with the answers she needed, her plight was hopeless. Although she used words to veil her intentions, it was clear she had made a decision to end her life.

The response was immediate, and members pleaded with her not to commit suicide. For one week posts were sent to her, with no reply. Then one came signed by her son. The woman had indeed tried to take her own life. Fortunately, her son had found her before it was too late. Because her computer had been left on, he had been able to read his mother's posts since the time of his father's death. He had had no idea of the amount of pain she was in. Fortunately, she recovered, is in counseling, and occasionally posts, but she no longer asks questions about how to regain her happiness.

There are in fact groups that are both supportive and informative, and this is the sort of group I most recommend. For example, see Memory People, for those in the Alzheimer's community, their caregivers, and advocates. The Open to Hope site contains a wealth of information and support for people attempting to get through grief. For men at any stage of prostate cancer, there's the Advanced Prostate Cancer group. For people with any type of pulmonary illness, there is the Chronic Obstructive Pulmonary Disease Foundation. As one caregiver said to me, "There is comfort in knowing that other people are experiencing the same things I'm going through." The members on some sites develop a virtual caring community and offer heartfelt condolences and practical guidance, and even say good night to caregivers who are alone. Social media groups can also provide an opportunity for you to help others. There may be aspects of your caregiving that differ from those of others. Your knowledge may help those struggling with what you have already solved. While medical advice is off-limits on some sites, others relate experiences their loved ones have had with various medications and procedures. The level of sophistication of medical advice ranges from "I heard on the *Larry King* show" to clinical research that some group members have personally conducted.

When exploring the various sites, follow the posts for at least one week. By then you'll have a good idea of which ones are sites for support, for information, for venting, or simply for the development of camaraderie between people experiencing the same thing as you. Rarely have I found a site that was harmful. The main problem is expecting the site to offer something it can't deliver.

WHEN YOU CAN NO LONGER CARE FOR YOUR LOVED ONE

There may come a time when, despite your wanting to care for your loved one, it may not be possible. Either you're physically unable or the emotional strain on you has become unbearable. You may need outside help to come into your home, or you may need to place a loved one in a care facility. It's a difficult decision, especially when a loved one pleads to remain at home or to be cared for only by you. But doing either might endanger him and be so punishing for you that you are no longer able to competently serve him.

I've often heard the phrase "I'll never put her in a nursing home" as a generic condemnation of all care facilities. While many facilities deserve the terrible reputations they have, others provide wonderful care. Many people believe that the more expensive the facility, the greater the likelihood that care will be outstanding. However, the cost of services is not always an indication of their quality. I served a woman at a small, inexpensive nursing home with staff so caring that

I would have felt comfortable being placed there. I've also been in expensive assisted living facilities where the selection of staff didn't match the scrutiny given to choosing the furniture.

So how do you decide on a facility? Recommendations are always helpful, but are often based on limited knowledge. A friend's loved one may have had a wonderful experience in a certain nursing home ten years earlier. But the likelihood that the same staff are still there is remote. There are two different approaches you can use for selecting a facility. The first involves the thought "I want the very best there is for my loved one, regardless of the cost." For someone with substantial financial resources or generous insurance coverage, this is an appropriate guiding principle. But for most people, the cost of an "ideal" care facility can be out of reach, especially if their funds or Medicare reimbursements are limited. For them, the question is: "Of all the facilities I can afford, which offers the best care for my loved one?"

Questions for Selecting Facilities and Services

Usually, by the time a loved one needs to be placed in a facility, the situation is critical. He may have become a danger to himself or to you, or you may no longer be able to physically or emotionally deal with his needs. It's often a time of desperation, when your overriding concern is whether someone will take your loved one. Decisions in that urgent situation are often based on what's available, not on what's best. To avoid making a crisis decision, you can do two things. First, explore what's available in your area long before you need to make a decision, even if you're convinced you'll never place your loved one in a care facility. What is unimaginable today may be a necessity tomorrow. Second, ask specific questions of the facilities you think you might consider. A great source of general questions relating to quality and safety can be found at Medicare.gov (www .medicare.gov/nursing/overview.asp). Although the site specifically discusses nursing homes, I believe most of the questions are appropriate for all care facilities. In the following list, I've supplied two sets of supplemental questions to ask. Professionals, family caregivers, managers of reputable facilities, and patients who experienced both great and less than adequate care suggested these questions to me. The first set is for both stand-alone facilities and home services. The second is just for stand-alone facilities.

Questions for Both Home Services and Stand-Alone Facilities

- Are you licensed by the state and/or a national association?
- Are your employees bonded?
- Has a background check been run on every employee?
- Can I see the background check of the person(s) who will be assigned to my loved one?
- How much training do your caregivers have?
- Have there been any complaints against your agency or employees, and if so, how were they resolved? (This information is available from your state-licensing agency.)
- Are your employees required to seek continuing education?
- What services can my loved one expect, and how often will they be given?
- What is the total monthly cost?

Questions for Stand-Alone Facilities

- Do you have any special certifications (for example, for caring for patients with Alzheimer's)?
- What is your staff turnover rate?
- What is your ratio of *caregiving* staff to patients?
- Do you have any formal relationships with hospice organizations?
- What is it about your facility that makes it stand out from others?

It may be uncomfortable to ask these questions. But reputable agencies and facilities will understand why you're asking them. If you meet resistance, the resistance itself may indicate problems the agency or facility might not want to disclose.

Even if it is too early to initiate a hospice service, it might be beneficial to contact one. Many hospice services offer homecare services, and even if they don't, they can probably provide you with a list of homecare agencies their patients have used. The advantage of using a hospice's homecare personnel is that, if your loved one must transition to a hospice, staff will already be familiar with him and you.

The Range of Placements

A wide range of placements is available for your loved one, and these different placements are designed to accommodate various stages in her illness. Some, such as assisted living, provide services throughout the illness. Others, such as skilled nursing, may focus only on a specific phase. The information in this section is derived from many federal and state sources and private facilities. Since there is great variation in state requirements and ongoing changes in federal regulations, more up-to-date information should be obtained directly from the agency or facility you are interested in.

Assisted living facilities provide help with the activities of daily living, like bathing, dressing, and using the bathroom. They may also help with the care most people do for themselves, such as taking medicine, using eyedrops, making appointments, and preparing meals. Residents often live in their own rooms or apartments within a building or group of buildings and have some or all of their meals together. Social and recreational activities are usually provided. Some of these facilities have health services on site. In most cases, residents pay a regular monthly rent and then pay additional fees for the services they receive. Medicare doesn't pay for assisted living facilities. The term *assisted living* may mean different things in different facilities. Not all assisted living facilities provide the same services.

Program of All-Inclusive Care for the Elderly (PACE) is unique. It is an optional benefit under both Medicare and Medicaid that focuses entirely on older people who are frail enough to meet their state's standards for nursing home care. It features comprehensive medical and social services that can be provided at an adult day health center, home, or inpatient facility. The comprehensive service package permits most patients to continue living at home while receiving services. PACE enrollees must

- be at least fifty-five years of age;
- live in the PACE service area;
- be screened by a team made up of a doctor, nurse, and other health professionals certifying they meet the state's nursing facility level of care; and
- be able to safely live in a community setting.

Social managed care plans provide the full range of Medicare benefits offered by a standard managed care plan. They also offer additional services such as coordination of services; prescription drug benefits; chronic care benefits covering short-term nursing-home care; and a full range of home- and community-based services, such as homemaker services, personal care services, adult day care, respite care, and medical transportation. Other services that may be provided include eyeglasses, hearing aids, and dental benefits. Whether Medicare pays for the social managed care plan depends on whether the patient meets eligibility criteria, which may include location, additional costs, and type of illness. At the time of this writing, plans were available only to individuals living in Portland, Oregon; Long Beach, California; Brooklyn, New York; and Las Vegas, Nevada.

Each plan has different premium amounts, and all plans have copayments for certain services.

Nursing homes serve as permanent residences for people who are too frail or sick to live at home or at temporary facilities during recovery periods. The number of residents in such a facility is usually small, with the maximum number set by your state. Medicare generally doesn't cover long-term stays in a nursing home. When loved ones live in a nursing home, they can still use Medicare coverage to pay for hospital care, doctor visits, and prescription drugs. It is important to compare the care that different nursing homes give, in order to decide which one will be best for your loved one. One way to do this is to look at the information about nursing home quality on a nursing home comparison website. Visit www.medicare.gov and select "Nursing Home Compare" (or go directly to www.medicare.gov/NH Compare). Nursing Home Compare's Five Star Quality Rating System is designed to give you easy-to-use information to help you choose a nursing home, to give you information about the care in nursing homes, to help you talk to nursing home staff about the quality of care, and to know the home's quality improvement efforts.

Skilled nursing facilities are nursing homes reimbursed by Social Security and Medicare. To be eligible for care by a Medicare-covered skilled nursing facility, a physician must certify that the beneficiary needs daily skilled nursing care or other skilled rehabilitation services that are related to the hospitalization, and that these services, as a practical matter, can be provided only on an inpatient basis. Services may be offered in a freestanding or hospital-based facility and covered by Medicare, Medicaid, or a long-term-care insurance policy.

Adult family homes in some states are an alternative to skilled nursing facilities when there is a wide range of services that can be delegated to a registered nurse. Such a home is a cross between a nursing home, where staff can administer limited medical procedures, and a skilled nursing facility that offers more services than a loved one might need. The homes are licensed for a small number of adults. With skilled providers, some homes can do intravenous infusion, wound therapy, wound care, and so on. When appropriate, hospice services can be provided by an independent agency. Adult family homes are also called "adult group homes" and "adult care homes." As in the case of nursing homes, each state has its own criteria for licensing.

Hospice care is a special way of caring for people who are terminally ill with six months or less to live. Under certain circumstances, best discussed with the hospice agency, the six-month requirement may be flexible. Hospice care includes physical care and counseling. The goal of hospice care is to provide comfort for terminal patients through pain management, not to cure the illness. As part of hospice care, your loved one will have a team of doctors, nurses, home health aides, social workers, counselors, and trained volunteers to help him and your family. Medicare covers hospice care if your loved one qualifies. Depending on his condition, he may get hospice care at home or in a hospice facility, hospital, or nursing home. Medicare doesn't cover room and board, nor does it pay for twenty-four-hour assistance if you get hospice services at home.

FINAL THOUGHTS

Long-term caregiving, especially for a loved one, may be one of the most difficult things you'll ever do. It also has the potential to be one of the most rewarding. Tibetans say, "You can't have tea without leaves, or meat without the bone." Similarly, the pain of rejection may accompany the joy you will experience from caring for a loved one. If you perceive the sharp points as being directed against you, your value as a caregiver will be compromised. It's been my experience that illnesses affecting the loved one's cognition or personality have the greatest negative effect on caregivers. It's difficult for someone who has sacrificed his life for the care of a loved one to be the recipient of abuse, even though he knows it's the illness talking. Understanding that the unskillful words of your loved one are just an inappropriate means of expressing her physical and emotional pain will do much to protect you. Let your loved one's expressions of pain slide off you; don't take them as an indictment against you. Vindictive words and actions whose source is a chronic or terminal illness are rarely about you. Your nonjudgmental acceptance is the price you'll pay for caring deeply about a loved one.

The future is always in a state of flux. What you may now believe to be unthinkable may be a necessity in the future, especially when it concerns the placement of a loved one. The earlier you prepare for the worst, the more comfortable you'll be if it happens, and the more delighted you'll be if it doesn't.

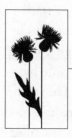

CHAPTER 3

Your Loved One's World

*I*magine being dropped into a strange country with a language you don't understand and customs that are unfamiliar. I experienced this when I was in Prague and decided to drive to Weimar, a four-hour trip. I didn't speak any Czech, and my German was as inadequate as it was when I studied it in high school. But I did have a GPS that guided me. Without the GPS, I probably would still be wandering around Germany. Your loved one is on a similar journey, but without a GPS. As the illness progresses, he will move into uncharted territory. He may have access to information about the illness, even about how to prepare for his own death. But all of that is still theory. What he is experiencing, both physically and emotionally, may be light years away from what publications say he *should* be feeling.

PERCEPTIONS

In the 1950s movie *Rashomon*, written and directed by Akira Kurosawa, four characters describe a gruesome death. Although the four had witnessed the same event, their descriptions of what happened were substantially different. Many people would reject the possibility that all four were telling the truth. After all, they all were involved in the same event and heard, touched, smelled, and saw the same things. But "truth" in the movie — and in caregiving — starts to change when information is crunched into something that goes beyond observation. Say, in another example, two people are listening to a Thelonious Monk CD. The first person, whose favorite musician is Lawrence Welk, hears discordant, random notes. The second person is a professional jazz musician who hears an incredible tune embellished by wonderful chords. The same event, but very different perceptions.

As you try to understand your loved one, think about why he is modifying information and experiences. It doesn't make much sense to talk about an independent reality that's the same for both of you. Unique filters continually shape everyone's experiences in accordance with their needs, fears, and beliefs. Say the physician talks about the minor changes in walking that will be necessary as your loved one's muscular strength diminishes: You hear information about what you'll need to do to compensate for living in a two-story house. Your loved one hears that his life is over.

The Power of Pain and the Fear of Death

Sometimes a loved one's behaviors are shaped by the effects of a chronic or terminal illness. What she hears and sees may have little to do with what you said or did. The ability to think and act in predictable ways can be affected by changes in metabolism, pain, or the realization that, until she dies her mind and soul will be occupying a shell she doesn't particularly like. In my hospice work, I've watched the physical effects of a brain tumor change a calm, peaceful man into a paranoid, aggressive person. Conversely, I watched someone who had practiced meditation throughout his life minimize the pain he was experiencing as his cancer metastasized. I've never had a client or patient who chose to be moody or to act irrationally. It's easy for a caregiver to become frustrated or confused when a loved one engages in bizarre or destructive behavior or shows no appreciation for a caregiver's sacrifices. There's always a cause. Sometimes it's related to perceptions, redefinitions of self, efforts to function in a world perceived as becoming increasingly chaotic, or unmet needs as the illness ravages mind and body.

Don't Argue about What's True

You may be tempted to argue with your loved one that her interpretation of what she heard or experienced was not "real," or that she is overreacting to a situation. Corrective suggestions, such as telling her what she should feel, rather than accepting what she does feel, are not productive. You're telling her that, despite the effects of her illness, her perception of the world should match yours. It doesn't, and it can't.

When I was a professor at San Francisco State University, I routinely did demonstration therapy in our communicative disorders clinic. One young woman I treated had recovered most of her speech and language functioning after she had a stroke. To someone who didn't know her, there were no outward signs that her ability to organize the world was compromised, but it was. "Maybe I should wear a sign," she said, "something like: My Brain Is Fried." She went on to tell me that her friends who were not chronically ill continually interacted with her based on how they thought she should experience the world. They would choose restaurants that were noisy, because, for them, noise meant this was a "happening place." Noise for my client meant an evening of confusion, frustration, and humiliation when she would pleasantly look at someone who was speaking, smile, nod her head, and have no idea what was being said.

We can argue with a loved one that his interpretation of what he heard or experienced wasn't real, or we can adapt what we are doing to meet his needs. The first approach may be fruitless and do little more than reduce the trust we so desperately need to maintain as the illness progresses. Or we can accept the reality of his interpretation and send him the explicit message that expressions of how he feels are legitimate.

Help Loved Ones Remain in the Most Comfortable Time Frame

How people view chronic and terminal illnesses is inherently tied to loss and time — what one had, what one will lose, and what will never occur. For some people, time frames shift almost effortlessly from the past to the present to the future in ways that are less than orderly. They can be connected by actions or thoughts. One patient insisted on driving a car even though he was susceptible to blackouts. Driving connected him to a time in the past when he was healthy. While thoughts that connect time to specific periods may not be dangerous, they can be confusing to someone listening to them.

That was the case with Hank. My visits would usually begin with him telling me how the week went. Within a few minutes he might begin talking about backpacking and fishing in Yosemite National Park, something he had done sixty years ago. Without any transitional thoughts, he might then lament the fact that he was no longer able to drive his truck, and then remember a time when he was a child playing stickball with neighborhood kids in Brooklyn. Once during a conversation about his occupation as a shoe salesman, he gave me an old trail map he had used for trekking and made me promise to take it on a trip to Yosemite that I had planned. There was never a logical order in what he chose to talk about; one time frame triggered another, often without my understanding why. And as in the case of the trail map, he often tried to link time periods together in ways I couldn't understand.

But some people, unlike Hank, do get stuck in a moment of time. It can be the past, present, or future. For Mary, it was the past. She had been instrumental in changing the lives of economically poor children through an after-school reading program. As her disease painfully progressed, she focused on her past accomplishments to make the present tolerable. In her mind, she had made a difference in the world; there was no need to regret not having a future; and the present, with its discomfort, was no match for the joy she experienced just by remembering the past. Other patients, like Eric, stayed in the present. He was dying from pancreatic cancer, had been divorced twice, had a history of drug problems, and never seemed to be able to hold a job for very long. But despite all his past tragedies, he had an eighteen-year-old son who was devoted to him. According to Eric, his son's love was sufficient for easing his death. For others, who live in the future, death comes much too early, regardless of their age or past accomplishments. That was the case with an author who had made significant contributions to the field of journalism and was widely published. He found no solace in what he had done, although he had a list of important publications that would have been the envy of any writer. With only days left to live, he kept looking for a manuscript.

"I have to finish it," he said to me. "It's due on Saturday. What day is it?"

"Tuesday," I said.

"Tuesday? How many days until Saturday?"

"Four."

"Four days! I have six chapters to complete. I need to find it *now*." He tried to get out of bed, but was too weak to sit up by himself. Another volunteer and I gently eased him back down.

"We'll find it for you, Bill," I said.

We kept searching the room until he fell asleep, but we couldn't find anything that even resembled a manuscript. Two days later he died. And as was the tradition in the hospice, staff, volunteers, and a few friends sat next to the body, and each talked about the impact Bill had made on our lives. I asked one of his friends about the manuscript.

"What manuscript?" a woman who had known him for many years said.

"Bill said he needed to finish a manuscript by Saturday."

"There is no manuscript. Bill hasn't written anything longer than a short article in ten years."

For this gifted writer, I don't think there could ever have been enough accomplishments. His desire to finish a nonexistent manuscript might have symbolized his not having completed enough of his goals. Being stuck in a specific time frame, or effortlessly migrating back and forth, is a result of experiences, values, and needs. For Mary, nothing could compare with a specific era in her past, and the longer she stayed there during our conversations and her thoughts, the happier she was. For others, like Bill, life was future oriented. But for many of my patients, residing firmly in the present resulted in an easier death. In the present they could let go of the past and relinquish the future. Changing how one lives close to the end of life is possible, but difficult. Sometimes the only thing you can do is be supportive of a loved one who has chosen to reside in the past or future.

Receiving Little or No Gratitude

Gratitude is a public statement of personal need. The grateful loved one is saying, "I can't do it anymore by myself." For many people, difficulty expressing gratitude, even to a caregiver, is not a sign of inconsiderateness. Rather, it can be a denial of their condition. Bruce, a retired educator, came to a hospice facility in San Francisco where I was a bedside volunteer. He had congestive heart failure and was obsessively independent. As he became weaker, Irma, a very considerate staff person, tried to serve him. He not only refused all her efforts but also often yelled at her. Allowing anyone to help him meant he was dying, something he couldn't accept, even though he was in a hospice facility. Once, after being screamed and cursed at, Irma quietly said, "I know you don't want my help now, but I want you to know, when you can accept it I'll be here for you."

Being grateful means that loved ones have accepted their new dependent status. For some, it comes easy. But for others, it's a long, painful process.

The Role of Spirituality and Religion

Spirituality is often confused with religion. It's been my experience that spirituality is one component of an easier death, and it can be found within or outside of religion. It's easy defining religion — you just refer to self-identifying labels such as Catholic, Baptist, Muslim, Jewish, Buddhist, and Presbyterian, to name a few. Spirituality is different. There are as many definitions of it as there are writers who try to explain it. For me, it's simply a feeling expressed by my patients about the connectiveness of people or about being part of something "bigger" than they are. One lesson I learned about the role of spirituality is that, although it is probably one of the most important elements in easing someone's death, often it's not enough, as was the case with Stu.

Stu was a devout Catholic who, until he became ill, attended Mass daily and believed in the power of confession and absolution. However, he had done something to a person (he never said who or what it was) that weighed heavily on him as he approached his death. "I know God has forgiven me. Father Joe made that clear. But it's not enough. I know she never will." Not being forgiven by the person he hurt haunted him until his death. The pain of not being forgiven and other regrets often trump spirituality whether or not it is associated with religious doctrine. Reinforce a loved one's spirituality, but understand that it may not be enough to ease his death.

Help Loved Ones Maintain Control

Imagine for a moment your life is negatively affected by people, objects, and activities. It may be an abusive boss, a landlord intent on evicting you, or a car that constantly breaks down. While these are oppressive, you could act to alleviate the situation. You could move on to another job, find a new apartment, or use public transportation. But what if none of these choices resulted in acceptable consequences? If you quit work, you might not find another job in this difficult economy. If you gave up your apartment, you might become homeless. If you couldn't afford to repair or replace your car, and no public transportation was available, you'd be stuck in your neighborhood. A lack of control would, at the very least, make you disagreeable.

Your loved one is in a much worse position. People who live with chronic or terminal illnesses constantly experience a lack of control, which often becomes more intense as the illness progresses. A patient of mine with advanced COPD knew that, without proper medication and the constant use of oxygen, he'd die. "I hate using the oxygen, it dries out my nose. And I hate the effect of the medicines on my bowels. But what am I going to do? I can't really choose not to use them. Doing that means I die."

Loved ones may have lost the ability to control some of the most fundamental aspects of their lives. But there are other things, maybe not as important, that they can still control. When I'm with patients, I routinely give them choices. Few may seem important to those whose lives are not disintegrating. But taken together, they still can result in the feeling "Yes, I can make choices about how I'll live out the rest of my life." The choices I offer are all simple:

"What would you like for lunch?"

"Shall I place the flowers over by the window, or would you like them closer?"

"When would you like me to visit next week?"

"Do you want any visitors today?"

These may seem like minor decisions when compared with the greater issues involved in chronic and terminal illnesses, but they're not. Imagine you have a pothole on your road that you can't avoid hitting each day when you leave your house. The county is bankrupt, so there's no money to fix it. You take the initiative and buy a bag of asphalt and fill the hole in order to save the shock absorbers on the car. You didn't fix the pothole, just rendered it less destructive. Giving choices to loved ones instead of making decisions for them, even with the most inconsequential things, throws a little more asphalt into that pothole.

When given choices by caregivers, loved ones feel they are being treated as if they still are intact human beings with desires, needs, and the cognitive ability to control some aspects of their lives. In the case of Alzheimer's or other illnesses affecting cognition, giving choices early on may be especially important as the illness progresses and cognitive ability is continually lost. Of course, as cognition becomes more impaired, the choices should only be ones that aren't potentially harmful, such as "Do you want eggs or cereal for breakfast?"

Sit When Talking

It is natural to stand when we visit someone who is in bed. What we don't realize is that we unintentionally convey a message of inequality: one person is standing up, looking down, while the other is supine, peering up. But if you sit on a chair so that you're both at the same eye level, the interaction often becomes one of equals.

I never saw the wife of one of my patients sit next to her husband in my presence. Their relationship had always been very formal, not only physically but also, according to their daughter, emotionally. The husband knew he was dying but was afraid to discuss it with his wife, because then she would know. The wife didn't want to talk about it with her husband, because then he would realize he was dying. I spoke to each individually and implied that possibly the other suspected what each already knew. I suggested that the wife take my seat next to her husband (I always sat when I visited) as I left to do an errand in another part of the house. I hoped that sitting next to her husband would make it easier for her to initiate the discussion. When I returned, they were holding hands and both were crying. Probably one of the most important discussions they ever had was stimulated by the act of sitting. I think sitting next to a loved one has the potential to change a relationship.

WHEN LOVED ONES MUST REDEFINE THEMSELVES

How we view ourselves — our identity — is based on what we do, the roles we play, the activities we enjoy, our affiliations, our abilities, our relationships, and the values that structure our lives, to mention only some of the multitude of things that constitute identity. All these in combination are used by loved ones to create a picture of who they are, and by other people as they anticipate reacting to them. When an integral part of a loved one's identity changes, so does her self-perception and place in the world.

Accept Feelings of Loss

Losing something that gives meaning to life is often a by-product of chronic and terminal illnesses. It can be the daily jog for someone who has run for forty years, the loss of hearing for someone who has played the cello her entire life, or the gradual memory loss of a writer who has spent his days in front of a computer crafting short stories. Most people can look at these losses and understand how devastating they are. But what about something like the inability to knit experienced by someone with crippling rheumatoid arthritis?

Or the inability to read the morning newspaper over a cup of coffee as one's eyesight diminishes?

Unfortunately, the magnitude of a loss is often thought of in terms of someone else's sense of what's important. An active person might think that no longer being able to walk is tragic, and the inability to knit inconsequential. Yet for someone with rheumatoid arthritis whose entire life centered on knitting, the loss is far more devastating then being unable to walk. Many chronic and most terminal illnesses result in life-changing losses. People's ability to knit, run, walk, write, or converse may disappear, but memories of these things remain constantly present, sometimes acting as slaps in the face when ailing individuals see others doing such things.

Caregivers try to be supportive by presenting "but look" arguments. "Yes, I know you can't jog anymore, *but look* at what you're still able to do." How convincing can that argument be when the activity or ability now lost was a central feature of a person's life? Ask anyone who has undergone a significant loss what she thinks about "but look" propositions. The head knows that it makes sense to relish what one is still capable of doing, but the heart mourns the loss.

We get enjoyment and fulfillment not from the thing, activity, or person itself but from the emotions it stirs in us. For example, I did solo wilderness fly-fishing throughout my adult life. It was the most enjoyable activity I ever did. When my cancer treatments and a chronic sleep disorder prevented me from continuing that pursuit, I mourned its loss as if it were a loved one who died. My head knew that I was fortunate that one group of medications was containing the cancer and another was allowing me to sleep. And not going into the wilderness alone was a small price to pay for sleep and life. But my heart still longed to go. I eventually realized that it wasn't the act of fishing in the middle of a pristine river that I missed; it was the serenity I felt being there. When I realized that, I sought other activities that could engender the same or a similar feeling. I found it in playing and crafting wooden flutes. Was it the same? Not really. But it allowed me to partially fill that pothole.

When your loved one laments the loss of something important, avoid using a "but look" response. The regret he's expressing is coming from the heart, and it needs a heart response. Begin exploring what made that activity so important in his life. Once the emotions have been identified, jointly think about what other activities *may* generate similar ones. Often the answer is found in very different activities, like when I found that playing and crafting flutes would substitute for wilderness fly-fishing.

As your loved one's illness progresses, you may find that what works today will not work tomorrow. Look for something that may be doable throughout his disease progression. If both of you realize that what he has chosen will be possible for only a short period of time, still do it, but think about what can substitute for it at a later point. For example, an ALS patient I served loved ambling through Golden Gate Park in San Francisco. He lived only a few blocks away and, before he was diagnosed, spent hours there every day. As the disease progressed and he no longer could walk, I would take him to the Rose Garden each week in his wheelchair. When he was confined to a bed, people who visited would come with a flower they picked from the park. Any loss that a loved one tells you is substantial, by definition is. Accept it as so and jointly explore substitutes.

Allow Loved Ones to Set the Pace of Increasing Dependence

As illnesses progress, loved ones may gradually lose different aspects of independence. Reduced independence is measured not only by physical activities but also by emotions. The abhorrence some people express about wearing absorbent briefs or using a catheter doesn't just involve physical discomfort: the thing they abhor is an undeniable sign they are getting closer to becoming incapacitated. The balance point between being helpful and aiding someone's independence constantly shifts. Becoming aware of it can allow you to be helpful without being solicitous.

When I was caring for my brother-in-law during the initial stages of his brain tumor, he did some dangerous things, such as insisting on walking without a cane or walker. He finally agreed to use both after coming to terms with his limitations. I've found that accepting a new, diminished capacity is a problem for many people, regardless of the illness. Often a frank, compassionate discussion of what a person is denying can change his behavior or, if not, at least allow the caregiver to understand why his loved one chooses to do something that may hurt himself or others. For my brother-in-law, walking unassisted had nothing to do with getting from one place to another. Rather, it was an expression of his independence.

I've found that when working with seniors, people recently disabled, or those with a chronic or terminal illness, it is sometimes futile to try to convince them not to do certain things. When that happens, try an alternative approach. Find out why your loved one insists on doing something she knows has potentially harmful consequences. When I was being treated for prostate cancer and was weak, I frightened my family when I insisted on taking a solo wilderness fly-fishing trip to the High Sierra. It wasn't that I didn't know what I was risking, but that my need to hold on to a part of my identity seemed important enough to outweigh my good judgment and concern for my family's feelings.

One of the hardest things for a person with a progressive disease to accept is a developing disability. The people I've served constantly struggled to balance their desire to feel independent with their realization that they needed help. "Should I offer to help?" a confused caregiver asked me. "Will she think I don't believe she can do anything? And if I offer help, am I implying that I think she's doing worse than she thinks?" Acceptance of a disability is a complicated matter. It's not just the willingness to go from independence to dependence but also the acceptance of the reality that you are becoming a different person.

One client said to me that in the beginning of his ALS, friends would hover over him as if he had already lost control of his arms and legs. "It was a difficult discussion for all of us, but we had a meeting where I told everyone that I knew I would eventually lose control of my muscles, but that, for the time being, there were many things I still could do. And I wanted to do as much as I could, for as long as I could. Did I need help? Of course. But, I said, 'Let me tell you when, and what I need.'"

Being overly helpful may require a loved one to accept his chronic or terminal illness before he is ready. Allowing too much independence may come across as being uncaring and, in some cases, may be dangerous. The best approach is to follow your loved one's lead. Ask him to let you know what he needs and what he can still do by himself. If you notice a reluctance to ask for help, it's time to have an honest discussion — one in which you focus not on his denial but on how the behaviors that are jeopardizing his safety frighten you.

Accept and Support New Identities

When I was teaching, it was always: "I'm a university professor." After I left teaching because of a chronic sleep disorder, it was: "I'm retired"; but I would quickly add: "I used to teach at the university." It was difficult for me to give up my role as a university professor since it was a large part of my identity. It wasn't just a title; I had fully lived the part. I made sure I didn't pepper my conversations with curse words or ungrammatical constructions. I didn't inappropriately scratch myself in public. My conversations were intelligently framed, and my behaviors were fitting of an educator. Then almost overnight, I was no longer a professor.

When roles are eliminated or modified because of illness, a loved one's view of the world and her place in it changes. The stripping away of something that gave meaning to life inevitably brings up the existential question "Who am I?" And even if the loss is anticipated, as in a lengthy illness, the actual change in roles is usually quick. A woman with ALS whom I served had been a powerful executive for fifteen years, and in a few months' time she became someone who relied on others for even the most basic needs. Almost everything she had built her life on was gone. There was nothing she could do to bring back the prestige she lost when she was forced to leave her position. But she could manage those who were responsible for her care. Each day, she would construct an assignment sheet; there, the responsibilities of each person, including me, were clearly specified. My job was to help her organize a family tree that went back to eighteenth-century Germany. Some of her friends couldn't understand why she was so demanding when they were only trying to help. What they didn't realize was that she was attempting to hold on to a disintegrating identity.

Accept and Support Unintended Consequences without Glorifying Them

It's not unheard of for a chronic or terminal illness to lead to unintended positive consequences. I would never say that developing prostate cancer was worth the lessons I learned from the illness. But I don't think that, without the illness, I would have developed the reverence I have for living in the present. Others, such as my former patient Ida, expressed similar thoughts. "Since the stroke," she said, "my relationship with my husband has never been better. There are people who felt uncomfortable with me after the stroke. We don't see them anymore, but the friends I have left are more precious to me than ever. I lost much after the stroke, but I've become more patient, I listen better, I don't take anything for granted — especially my health — and I live today like there is no tomorrow. Would these things have happened without the stroke? Probably not. But that doesn't mean I'm glad I had it."

Help Loved Ones Simplify Their Worlds

I was preparing for a thirty-day trip to Japan, where I would be tracing the history of the Japanese bamboo flute, or *shakuhachi*, and studying with master teachers, some of Japan's "national treasures." We would be traveling throughout the country by train, and our luggage was limited to what we could carry on our backs and hold in our hands. My decisions on what to take or leave behind would affect the quality of the trip. Too many items and the weight would be burdensome. Not enough of the right ones and I might be forced to neglect some basic needs.

We all make decisions of this type daily. Take what's important, leave behind what isn't. But we tend to be oblivious to the importance of these decisions to possibly the most momentous journey of our lives — our deaths. And when we choose wrongly, the burden can be, as it was for Joyce, oppressive. The first time I met Joyce she told me about her fellow teachers who had been incredibly cruel to her when she was thirty years old. For one hour I listened to a litany of abuse. Since Joyce was in her late seventies, what she was describing had happened more than forty years before. Every week for the next month, she told me the same story. During one visit she leaned back in her chair and softly said, "You know, dying is such hard work." For two months her physical condition had been steadily declining, and so I assumed she was referring to her pulmonary problems. She paused, and then said, "I'm not talking about what's happening to my body." Pointing to her head, she continued: "The hard work is what's happening up here." For Joyce, the reluctance to let go of what had happened in her past needlessly added more baggage than she could handle on her journey.

In some ways Joyce's reluctance to let go of her fellow teachers' cruelty is similar to stuffing a suitcase with more items than it was designed to hold. Although clothes are bulging out of the unclosed suitcase, you decide it can still hold one more item. You slip it in and, while pressing down as hard as you can, struggle to close the zipper. Although you are getting a very clear message that this might have dire consequences, you gloat, delighted that you won't have to carry along another suitcase. As you look at your overstuffed bag with admiration, you notice the zipper's seam is slowly letting go. When a loved one holds on to what is no longer necessary, it results in similar consequences. But what unravels is his ability to deal with his progressive illness.

Sometimes, the problem begins with a caregiver's inability to understand that, as her loved one's illness progresses, he can't deal with as many items as before. On a 1950s television show called *Dragnet*, two detectives would interview victims or witnesses, whom they would allow to ramble on and intersperse observations about what happened with possible motivations for the crime, as well as personal experiences having nothing at all to do with the crime. Eventually, one detective would say the show's most famous line: "All we want are the facts, ma'am, just the facts." Often we give loved ones more information than is necessary. Or, like the witnesses in *Dragnet*, we combine a series of messages, many of which have nothing to do with the most important one. As the illness progresses and your loved one's ability to focus on verbal messages becomes more impaired, it's important to streamline what you say. That doesn't mean withholding information but "adjusting" the amount you say and speed at which you deliver it. In chapter 4, you'll find practical suggestions for how to accomplish this.

Many of my patients experienced a stimulus overload as their illnesses progressed. It wasn't that they were dealing with more things. Rather, pain and fear of the future reduced their ability to focus on the same number of things at once. For example, the CEO of a multinational company had difficulty each morning deciding what

he would have for breakfast. A professor who had spent his life ana-
lyzing language had problems following simple conversations. A
carpenter who had built houses couldn't complete easy manual tasks
without becoming frustrated. None of these patients had dementia.
I believe the information-processing problem they had was related
to three factors: an abundance of issues requiring their attention, not
enough time to come to terms with them, and a diminished ability to
concentrate. Some of them coped by limiting the number of people
who could visit, although many relatives and friends misunderstood
their decision to do so. Other patients cut back or eliminated lifelong
interests to reduce the overload. And for some, not talking about
highly emotional issues was effective.

Many things that were important when a loved one was healthy
may no longer be of interest. As an illness progresses, many loved
ones focus on only those things that will make it less oppressive.
Often, when they try to maintain the interests they had before the illness, they experience a reduced focus on the more important things,
such as asking for forgiveness, expressing gratitude, and so forth.
Loved ones can't keep adding more things to think about without
this additional burden affecting the quality of their thinking.

Holding on to interests that are no longer relevant may also be
a person's attempt to deny the reality of her condition, or she may
do so for the benefit of friends and family who wish to keep alive the
fantasy that everything is just as it was before the diagnosis. I often
go to a remote cabin where I write. I don't make phone calls, I have
no Internet access, and I can't hear city traffic. Just as I'm able to
concentrate more on the writing there than in my office in San Francisco, people who are chronically or terminally ill are able to focus
more clearly when superfluous things are reduced or eliminated.
Help your loved one pare away activities irrelevant to her new life.
As a progressive illness continues to define who she is, help her simplify her life, enabling her to focus on what's important in accepting
her illness or death.

Shedding Defensiveness

When I was growing up in eastern Pennsylvania, with its bitter winters, my mother would dress me in layers of clothing to keep me warm during the routine single-digit January temperatures. When I returned from a morning of playing in the snow, she would peel the layers off: mittens, hat, scarf, snowsuit, sweater, and flannel pajamas. All the layers were necessary to ward off the cold outdoors. But once inside, they were superfluous. It's analogous to the world of the person who has a chronic or terminal illness. I found that, as illnesses progressed, layers of defenses that developed over a lifetime were gradually shed. Time is too short for mixed messages. Loved ones may have much they want to say and do when they realize they are getting closer to dying. When I hear the phrase "being an authentic person," I identify it with the transparency I see in adults as they prepare to leave.

That's what I saw in Guy's words and behaviors. He had been a firefighter in San Francisco before retiring. At seventy-five, he was in the last stage of lung cancer. "All my life I've been strong, both mentally and physically," he said. "I'd go with my crew into a burning building to do our primary search. I wasn't afraid of anything, not even the blowups." He paused as if rethinking what he'd just said. "If I was, I never showed it. We'd fight a fire for hours, my Nomex pants smoldering; and even when I was the 'old man' of the crew, I outdid firemen half my age. I was good. And when we would pull out bodies, especially kids, and wait for the bus, many of the guys who were fathers would be in tears, but not me. I would just do my job: reenter the building with the flame-over going full force. I never showed any emotions, no matter what I felt. Maybe that's why I couldn't find anyone to marry." He started to laugh, then abruptly stopped. "Believe me, pulling out kids tore me up, but I never showed it. Now, things are different."

"How?" I said.

"I don't feel I need to hide anything. You know, it's like I don't care what people think about me. I'm not trying to be the heroic fireman. None of that is important anymore. I'm afraid of dying, and I want to talk about it." He did over the next few weeks, often with tears flowing down his cheeks. Death is such a fundamental issue in a person's life that, when it is accepted, guards that have developed over a lifetime become superfluous.

FUNCTIONING

Despite the consuming nature of an illness, your loved one still needs to function. But the world he is functioning in has changed. The house that was a refuge from a chaotic world may now be a prison. The soft, comfortable bed, which may have been the scene of amorous nights, is now a reminder of what is no longer possible. The ambient noise of the street, which gave the neighborhood life, becomes a source of general agitation that affects even the most rudimentary thinking. Things have changed, and your loved one's ability to adapt will require your understanding and help.

Introduce Predictability

Most of us want predictability in our lives. If I buy an apple today, I expect that it will taste similar to the one I ate yesterday. When the traffic light turns green for me, I expect cars to my left and right to stop so I can go through the intersection without being hit. But what if the apple I eat today tastes like an onion? What if waiting for a red light to turn green before proceeding becomes optional? I probably would stop eating apples and would wait until no cars were present at an intersection before going through it, even when my light was green. But what if the unpredictability spread into other areas of my life? What if I knew that the absence of pain I felt today *might* be replaced by pain tomorrow? My distress would become uncontrollable and expressed in ways my caregivers might not understand. We may want some uncertainty and a bit of spontaneity to spice up our lives, but it's predictability that allows us to function sanely on a daily basis.

For many people with chronic and terminal illnesses, predictability may be elusive. One day, the pain of illness is controlled by medication or who knows what; the next day it comes on with the power of a sledgehammer. On good days, although there's reason for jubilation, there's also fear that the reprieve will end. On bad days, there's fear that the pain will persist and never relent. Certainty for many people with chronic or terminal illnesses is limited to the knowledge that the illness will continually progress, continually worsen. Figuring out what will help is often like hitting a moving target. A patient once said to me, "I don't know what tomorrow will bring. When I'm in pain, I pray that it'll stop. When it stops, I pray that the relief lasts. It's never knowing how long each will continue that's so difficult. If someone said, 'Marcy, you have a choice. You can either have six hours of pain followed by two hours of relief until you die, or one to three hours of pain followed by two to six hours of relief, but you'll never know in advance how much of each you'll experience,' I'd take the longer period of pain, because at least I'd know how long it and the relief would last."

You can make things more predicable by simplifying "if-then" relationships for loved ones. For example, when the alarm goes off, then it's time to get out of bed. When the mail arrives, then you and your loved one sit at a table and go through the material. If it's Tuesday morning, then it's time for a bath. These "if-then" propositions and hundreds of others may introduce an aspect of predictability that can help stabilize a loved one's life.

Focus on What Loved Ones Are Experiencing

There is uncertainty in disease progression, as well as in what happens as one begins to die, and afterward. Loved ones may have read numerous books, had a rigorous spiritual practice, and thought they were ready, only to find they are covering new territory. One patient even attended a weeklong workshop in which he simulated his own death. He left believing he had received a preview of what would happen. Two weeks before he died, though, he said, "What I experienced there has nothing to do with what I'm going through now." The great linguist Alfred Korzybski summarized the disparity between theory and reality: "The map is not the territory." What he meant was that there is an inherent difference between what we think something will be and what it is. This is theory and reality. As the end of life drew closer for many of my patients, what they thought was knowledge often was not. One patient described to me an interaction he'd had with his oncologist four years before coming to hospice.

My oncologist explained that treatment for my cancer would need to become more aggressive as the cells learned to adapt to the drugs. I sat calmly and asked the questions an "informed" patient should. I understood that this would be a holding action. That since the cancer cells had metastasized, the best we could hope for was to slow their growth, until a more permanent fix appeared. This was information, the core of life I always felt comfortable with. Every three months I visited him, and we had the same conversation, marveling for four years that our fight against the cancer cells was successful.

When I received the news that I knew was inevitable — the treatment protocol was losing its effectiveness and the cancer was growing — I didn't react as I had expected. Intellectually, for four years I had known the treatment would eventually fail. Shouldn't I have calmly accepted the news? Shouldn't logic have prevailed? Yes, to both, but neither occurred. I was in shock, even with the advance knowledge that this would happen.

It seems that knowing and experiencing, at least for my patient, resided in parallel universes. Your loved one will probably have a similar experience, but instead of years to contemplate the differences, as my patient had, she may have only months, weeks, or days. Just when she is adapting to a new physical or emotional phase of the illness, it may progress. Even having accurate information on what is occurring doesn't mitigate the feeling that death is one step closer. As I've learned with so many things in life, there is a difference between anticipating how you think you'll experience an event and how you actually do. When your loved one appears to have accepted the inevitable one day, and the next day expresses a great deal of fear, don't try to minimize it, unless the fear relates to something specific that you can explain — for example, to pain, the effects of certain drugs, and so on. She is telling you what she *is* feeling. Your good intention to minimize her fears can be misinterpreted if you tell her what she *should* be feeling. It's best to bear witness to her anxiety and be supportive.

Maintain Structure

Tibetans talk about internal and external *drahla*. *Drahla* is, essentially, a sense of order that one experiences. Creating internal *drahla* would involve eliminating thoughts that are not helpful for coming to terms with a chronic or terminal illness. For example, dwelling on what has been lost does little to facilitate acceptance of what is left. External *drahla* is the world that surrounds your loved one. A disorderly room filled with items related to an illness (such as medicines, absorbent briefs, and pads) focuses loved ones on the illness. An orderly room with a limited number of medical items, and with many objects related to past good memories, will enable your loved one to think more about the beauty of the life he experienced, rather than the dreadfulness of his illness.

When there is disorder — internal or external — I've seen families and health care staff misinterpret the behaviors that it generates. What they may consider to be a loved one's bizarre behaviors may be his attempts to regain the sense of structure that previously allowed him to map out what was familiar in his life.

A patient I served in his home was receiving excellent care from his wife and the hospice staff who regularly visited. But he complained that schedules were always changing. One week a nurse came on a Tuesday, the following week, a Wednesday. Although nobody ever missed an appointment, was terribly late, or provided anything less than exemplary care, the unpredictability of the visit days was unsettling to him. Sameness in scheduling introduces a small amount of predictability, which can reduce uncertainty.

Make Things Familiar

At a workshop I gave, one woman was perplexed that her husband became uncommunicative when she placed him in a nursing home. Regardless of what his wife said to him, he would sit in a chair and stare at the wall. She found it unsettling because one week before, while he was still in their home, he had communicated in short but intelligible phrases.

"I don't know what to do," she said. "He's so miserable. I can't care for him anymore at home, and I don't know what happened at the nursing home to cause the change."

"Describe for me what's in his room," I said. She proceeded to describe all the basic furniture that came along with the room. "And is there anything from home that he could relate to?" She said no. "What was his passion before becoming ill?"

"Golf. He lived for golf. Our living room is filled with trophies and pictures of him playing in tournaments."

"Then that's what I suggest you bring into his room. As many of the trophies and pictures as you can."

The following week she filled his room with trophies, pictures, and even his golf clubs. He again became responsive. Surround your loved one with objects, music, and smells that are familiar and peaceful. They can be pictures of people he cares about, favorite places, awards commemorating achievements, favorite objects, meditative music, or flowers. We know that memory is stored as fractured bits of information — visual images in one area, smells in another, and so on. By tapping into every aspect of a memory, it may be possible to bring it out even if one modality is damaged.

I recently served a professor emeritus of archaeology at an assisted living facility. When I entered his room, I saw that almost every flat surface and the walls were covered with mementos of his life, ranging from pictures and objects from archaeological digs to the leather caps he wore in the 1960s as a member of a notorious motorcycle club. When I sat next to him, he focused on one item, and as he weaved an engrossing story we were transported to a 1970s archaeological dig in Uganda. When we came back, he pointed to a picture of himself astride his Harley. "Let me tell you about that picture," he said, and off we went to an Oakland bar in the early 1960s as he confronted members of the Hell's Angels. What he had done was to create stability through familiar objects related to wonderful parts of his life. It's easy to do the same in your home or in any facility.

Make Learning New Behaviors Easy

As a chronic or terminal illness proceeds, your loved one may have to learn a new behavior. It may be a purely physical one, such as how to transition from a bed to a wheelchair. It may be cognitive, such as when to take daily medications. Or it may be emotional, such as how to reduce her anxiety as pain becomes uncontrollable. New behaviors have traditionally been taught in three ways. The first is by overlearning a specific behavior until it becomes automatic. For example, to transfer from bed to wheelchair, your loved one would continually practice the movement until she mastered it — usually just by moving from one location to another when it is necessary. Yes, eventually she will learn the movement, but only after some failures. However, even when the new behavior is learned, it often doesn't carry over to other activities, such as getting up out of a chair and onto a bed.

A second, more modern, approach is to use strategies for producing the behavior, rather than just practicing it. For example, I served a man with congestive heart failure whose physician had suggested he drink a certain amount of water four times each day. If he drank too little at one time, he would become dehydrated. Too much, and the water would be uncomfortably retained. He was never sure how much he drank. Usually, it was too much. I suggested that there be one bottle with lines drawn on the outside, along with the times he could drink. Those graphics became a strategy with which he was able to effectively monitor his water intake. We used a similar strategy (putting stickers on a clock) when he was supposed to move about his room.

A third way of making learning easier is to break down the new behavior into small units. I served a woman who lived in her own home and, because of financial difficulty, had limited caregiving. During the day, someone was there for up to four hours, but for the rest of the day and the night she was alone. When I came to see her one day, she told me it had been difficult to sleep because she had been cold. I checked the thermostat and saw that the control was turned to "off." At night when it had become too hot, she had turned off the heat rather than lowering the thermostat. I took a sheet of paper and wrote out the directions with graphics for what to do when she was hot and what to do when she was cold. Each step was numbered. For the next month the strategy worked beautifully, until her dementia progressed and she forgot to look at the sheet, even though it was still next to the thermostat. To adapt to her needs, I printed the instructions on a neon-yellow piece of paper. It was a strategy that worked until her dementia advanced to the point that she required constant care. The lesson for me was: whenever possible, always use a distinctive strategy, but understand what worked yesterday may not work today.

This step approach can even be used for something as ill-defined as the control of anxiety. One patient was trying, unsuccessfully, to meditate to control her anxiety between the time her pain developed and the time her medication became effective, which was about twenty minutes. I suggested that she use the technique for thirty seconds rather than the full twenty minutes — although this meant that for nineteen-plus minutes, until the medicine took the pain away, she would be anxious about it. She didn't understand the logic of my suggestion, but she tried it and was able to control her anxiety for a limited amount of time. Then, every time she needed the pain medication, her husband asked her to add an additional thirty seconds to her meditation. It took more than two weeks, but eventually she was able to keep her anxiety at a manageable level for the whole twenty minutes until her medication became effective.

Don't Assume It's Self-Centeredness

I'm sure self-centeredness is an explanation for the abuse some loved ones heap on their caregivers. But it's been my experience that inconsiderate behaviors are less about self-centeredness and more about a loved one coming to grips with his illness and eventual death. I spoke with a caregiver who attributed everything nasty her elderly father said to his lifelong self-centeredness. Although some of her examples could well have been a result of his belief that he was the center of the world, this became the first explanation she would go to when he became demanding. With his progressive heart failure, he gradually lost the ability to do many physical things. When he asked his daughter to hand him a box of tissues, and getting them himself would have required only a slight movement on his part, she became angry, since she was in the next room and he was within reaching distance of the box. Unfortunately, not having his current legitimate needs met caused him to escalate his demands. Eventually, his daughter felt she could no longer care for him. Despite his protests, she had him moved to a nursing home. As I heard this story, I wondered if the outcome would have been different if his daughter hadn't broadly identified most of his requests as stemming from self-centeredness.

Yes, there are some truly nasty people among those we care for. But starting with the belief that their cruelty comes from a prior narcissism that gets released with age or illness doesn't give us much to work with. We can either ignore these people's behavior or become angry with them. It's been my experience that bizarre and hostile behaviors are often related more to a fear of death, dependence, and infirmity than to self-centeredness. I've always found that, as my patients get closer to dying, their bizarre behaviors usually relate to things in their lives they haven't finished doing or to an inability to use traditional means of communicating. Helping them complete these issues, or learning how they communicate their needs, can be more effective than sedation or counseling. Look for legitimate explanations for what appear to be narcissistic behaviors. It's too easy to assume these unskillful behaviors are the result of self-centeredness.

But what about unskillful behaviors that were evident in certain loved ones long before they became ill? One caregiver said, "My mother has always been self-centered and egotistical. The only thing the dementia has done is increase it. I see no reason to give in to her cruelty." The daughter's solution was to ignore requests that she felt came from her mother's darker side. If only we could separate behaviors by their motivations that easily, caregiving would become more of a science than an art. If you start with the premise that some behaviors and requests are unreasonable, then most likely you will ignore many that are generated by the illness.

I've often found that there is an escalation of a loved one's unskillful words and behaviors when some are initially treated as if they were manufactured out of pre-illness needs. And when that occurs, resulting in caregivers continually experiencing psychological abuse, many believe they have few options other than placement in a facility. I'm speculating that some of the abuse may be a consequence of caregivers not accepting the legitimacy of behaviors that originate from the illness. This doesn't mean that acceptance always leads to pleasant outcomes or negates the need to place a loved one in a facility. Rather, acceptance can make a terrible situation less oppressive if caregivers understand that the criticism has nothing to do with them.

So the next time you are perplexed by the "ingratitude" or "hostility" of your loved one, don't assume she is being inconsiderate or thoughtless. It could be that you don't understand how her illness has shaped her words or behavior. You'll be amazed how far a little compassion and acceptance, and a lot of understanding, will go. Become a great Aikido martial arts master, if not to protect yourself, then to protect your loved one.

WHAT YOUR LOVED ONE NEEDS FROM YOU

People with chronic or terminal illnesses engage in a multitude of behaviors that caregivers don't understand. These may range from cleaning out cabinets in a garage that hasn't been touched in ten years to wanting a caregiver continually in attendance. Such behaviors are often expressions of need that, for whatever reason, can't be communicated through traditional means. Unfortunately, they are sometimes misidentified as emerging signs of psychosis.

I still vividly remember a black-and-white photograph of a young Sicilian boy taken by Richard Avedon in 1947. The boy was in the foreground of the photograph, smiling broadly and wearing a jacket that was too short in the sleeves and too tight in the chest. In the background, softly out of focus, stood a tree with a symmetrical oval canopy, and a fence that defined a boundary between the sky and the ocean. A seemingly bucolic scene unless you looked carefully at the boy. After staring at it for a while, I realized that the ill-fitting suit probably had little to do with parents who couldn't afford one that fit properly. The boy's body appeared to be racked with deformities: a back that appeared to be humped, emaciated legs, and a chest out of proportion to his body. My first impression of the photograph was clearly different after I looked at it carefully. Years after I saw the photograph, someone who understood Italian told me that the title of the photograph, *Noto*, was Sicilian for "dwarf." The figure in Avedon's photograph is analogous to behaviors of our loved ones that we may not understand. What we see initially may not reflect what is happening.

Acceptance and Respect

Jean, a hospice patient, refused to allow her mother to visit. Her mother was distraught, and some hospice staff and volunteers, including me, tried to convince Jean it would be healing to forgive whatever her mother did. She wouldn't even discuss it. And our insistence that she try transformed her trust in us to near-suspicion. During one delusional episode after that, close to the end of her life, she relived the last time her father had molested her while her mother sat in the living room pretending it wasn't happening. Behaviors — especially those we don't understand — are analogous to the pools of water that collect in marshes following a heavy rain. The water seeps into unseen deep holes that appear deceptively shallow. Relying on surface appearances places us at risk of misinterpreting other people's behaviors, as my fellow hospice workers and I did. Accept even what you may not understand, since many of the confounding things you will experience come from a world you may have been granted only limited access to.

After my fiasco with Jean taught me a lesson about the importance of acceptance, I made use of this invaluable information with

Bill. For two months, I spent every Friday with him. He was dying of hepatitis, and we would drive to Lands End, a scenic place in San Francisco, where we would sit on a bench and watch the Golden Gate Bridge, on our right, and the Pacific Ocean, on our left. As Bill smoked his medical marijuana to stop the nausea from his pain medication, he talked about his life. As much as I wanted to probe, I realized that it was important for him to tell his life history to someone who wouldn't judge him. I rarely asked questions. And when I did, it was only for clarification. His lifestyle was different than mine, and some of our values conflicted. But I tried not to be judgmental. At one of our last outings, he confided to me events that he had never told anyone. He said he shared them with me because, as terrible as they were, he needed to talk about them with someone who wouldn't judge him.

If Not Compassion, Then Understanding

Since progressive illnesses and dying are major events, we often believe that compassion needs to be expressed in big ways. It doesn't. Forget about big gestures and focus on expressing your love through the simplest of things, from the placement of flowers to sitting supportively in the presence of pain. When asked to define *compassion*, the Vietnamese Buddhist monk Thich Nhat Hanh said to think about how you would treat a person if he or she were your mother, the person who gave you life, fed you, and protected you. With that image in mind, being compassionate with some loved ones is as easy as breathing. Others, however, are less like the mother envisioned by Thich Nhat Hanh and more like the witch in *Snow White and the Seven Dwarfs*. Although I always tried to interact with patients as if they were my mother, occasionally an ogre materialized.

That was the case with Clarence. He was in his eighties and had lived most of his life in Alabama. He grudgingly moved to San Francisco to be with his daughter when he could no longer care for himself. With his view of blacks, Jews, Catholics, and "them damn agitators," he was the same as those who opposed the civil rights movement in the 1960s. As someone who was involved in the movement, whose parents were Jewish, and who was a lifelong "damn agitator," I stood for everything he hated. As much as I tried to use Thich Nhat Hanh's advice, I couldn't. Here was someone who may have been one of the people throwing stones at me as our bus arrived in Montgomery. Or he could have been the mounted policeman who was intent on making his horse stomp me as I cowered on the steps of the state capitol. Or possibly the jailer who ordered black prisoners to drag me and other white marchers from an integrated cell to a segregated one. Although he wasn't any of them, in my mind he represented all of them. He was dying and looked to me for compassion. And my convictions said, "Give it," but I couldn't.

There are times when, despite our best efforts, we can't become the person we want to be. I aspired to be compassionate to Clarence, to connect with him as a human being. I wanted to serve him, but I thought I couldn't. Then I realized that, when compassion couldn't be tapped into, understanding might be. What would I have become if I had been born in Selma to segregationist parents whose great-great-grandparents owned slaves, and whose fundamentalist religion espoused the superiority of whites, Protestants, and the Confederate cause? How different would I be? It was a matter of happenstance that I was born in the North to parents who were Jewish and who, because of the persecution they had experienced in Europe and the United States, taught me the importance of tolerance. Clarence, on the other hand, was born in a place with a history of bigotry. It was the circumstances of our lives that made us different. There may come a time during a loved one's care when his need for compassion isn't, in your mind, deserved. Instead of withholding it, try to understand his motivations for the unskillful things he has done. Try to understand the circumstances of his life.

Willingness to Listen to a Death Wish

I had been serving Bruce for more than two months when, during a period of intense psychological pain, I asked him if there was anything I could do to help. "Shoot me," he said. I waited for him to say something that would change the meaning of the words, but his plaintive stare continued, as did the words. "Shoot me, *please*." When I was finally able to compose myself, I said, "I can't." His eyes teared up and then they closed. Although Bruce was experiencing physical pain, I believe it was the psychological pain that led him to ask for my help. He had been a drug addict most of his life, was estranged from his family, and believed he was responsible for the death of his son. He felt that there would not be sufficient time for him to tie up the loose ends of his life, and therefore that his dying would be a painful psychological event. And he was right. As I sat at his bedside and watched the agony he was experiencing, I wondered what I would have done had he been my loved one and had I been more concerned about his pain than my own personal ethics or the laws of California.

What if your loved one asks you, pleads with you, to help him take his own life or, even worse, asks you to do it? I think it's more than hopelessness that can lead very ill people to wish they were dead. As one patient said to his wife, "I'm going to die no matter what you do, so why shouldn't I go out when things are still all right?" His concern was with the pain he expected to experience as his condition worsened. With advances in palliative care, pain reduction is possible, and when there is still discomfort, terminal sedation may be an option if strict medical criteria are met. Once sedation begins, all communication with a loved one ceases.

With terminal sedation, a loved one goes into a coma and, as long as the administration of sedation continues, remains in a coma until the illness takes its final course. I've known two patients who chose terminal sedation. One was a man with bone cancer who was allergic to morphine and all its derivatives. Before being sedated, he spent three days in unimaginable pain having his final conversations with his wife. Another was a man with ALS. Although he had no pain, he chose to be sedated when he no longer could move any part of his body.

Everyone approaches his or her death differently. My hospice patient who blamed himself for his son's death felt there was nothing he could do that would make his death any easier. The late Reverend Roshi Jiyu-Kennett, abbess of the Shasta Abbey Buddhist Monastery, viewed the pain she experienced near the end of her life differently. Before going to bed, one of the monks had the evening assignment of making sure she was comfortable. As her cancer progressed, she was in constant pain. According to the monk, as he left her room he heard her say something like: "Thank you, dear Buddha, for giving me one more day to perfect myself." Roshi Jiyu-Kennett looked at every day — especially those filled with intense pain — as an opportunity to become a better person.

Although palliative medicine can reduce physical pain, it often has little effect on psychological pain. I believe the emotional distress experienced by loved ones can be reduced by using the caregiver suggestions throughout this book. Using them may not prevent a discussion initiated by your loved one about hastening his death, but it can change your loved one's consideration of an early exit. Even if you apply every suggestion in this book, however, there may come a time when a loved one will still want to talk about taking his own life or will want you to assist him. That's not a time to talk about legalities, religious doctrines, or various ethical "shoulds." It's a time to listen, reflect, and realize he is grappling with probably the most important issue he has ever thought about. And you will be the one he has chosen to hear it. I've found that sometimes giving permission to a loved one to discuss a wish to die leads to an understanding of the psychological distress he or she is feeling, which is something you may be able to address.

FORMS GUARANTEEING YOUR LOVED ONE'S LAST WISHES WILL BE MET

There are few things that bring death to the forefront of a loved one's consciousness more readily than looking at documents addressing her last wishes. This chore may be so uncomfortable that most healthy people won't look at such a document until they enter a hospital and a social worker nonchalantly talks about a Do Not Resuscitate (DNR) order. When it happened to me, I was about to have surgery to remove my prostate, and the shock of reading the document minutes before I was about to walk into the surgical suite was horrific.

It is never too early to begin assembling documents that will assure that the wishes of a loved one will be honored when she no longer can express them. As of yet, no end-of-life legal document is acceptable in all states. The purpose of this section is to familiarize you with the five different forms available, but not to make any specific recommendations. In appendix 4, you can find where to obtain the forms. I encourage you to contact your attorney and learn what the legal requirements are for your state. Your loved one need not choose just one. For example, in California, many people file both a Physician Orders for Life-Sustaining Treatment (POLST) form and a DNR form.

If your loved one chooses to file one or more end-of-life documents, it's important that copies are provided to all those who may be involved with her care. This includes you, other family members, the hospital or care facility, physicians, other health care providers, and your attorney. During a medical emergency, the last thing you or the person caring for your loved one will want to do is search for a form. Some of these forms provide significantly overlapping information. Many people believe that redundancy is a good thing, and they use more than one form. In most states, if there is a difference between the wishes expressed in different documents, the document deemed most recent is honored. In choosing which one(s) to use, consider the following three things.

- How specific is the document? The greater the specificity, the more useful it will be.
- Is it legal? This is a straightforward question that an attorney can answer.
- Is it acceptable? Is this form known and accepted in the medical community?

Whatever form(s) you and your loved one decide to use, discuss it (or them) with each medical care provider, and, as noted earlier, supply each with a copy.

Medical Care Power of Attorney

With this document, your loved one appoints someone else to make decisions regarding his or her medical care when he or she is unable to do so. It's also called a Durable Power of Attorney for Health Care. This document is useful when a loved one can no longer communicate with others because of conditions ranging from incapacitating physical illness, such as degenerative heart disease, to cognitive problems, such as Alzheimer's. The person named in the Medical Care Power of Attorney will communicate for the patient. Most likely, this will be you. Your loved one can specify an alternate if for any reason you aren't available to make a decision. It's better not to ask two or more people to share this power of attorney equally. The last thing needed when a critical decision must be made quickly is a debate. Everyone needs to understand that the person named in the document has the ultimate decision-making power, even if others are consulted.

Although Medical Care Power of Attorney forms are easy to understand and execute, they are profound in what they imply. The person agreeing to accept the legal position may become responsible for continuing or ending a loved one's life. A decision of this type may be the hardest you'll ever have to make, even knowing that the choice you decide on is what your loved one would want you to do. That was the case with Ruth when she asked the hospital to withdraw all life support from her partner of twenty years, Giselle, who was in a vegetative state. Months before Giselle had had her final stroke, the two of them had talked about what Giselle wanted Ruth to do in the event of another, devastating stroke. When it occurred, Ruth had to make the painful decision to honor her partner's request. She did it in opposition to her partner's sister, who wanted to prolong Giselle's life as long as possible and threatened to get an injunction to stop the withdrawal of all life support. Without the document, the wishes of an estranged family member might have overruled Giselle's wishes.

Most Medical Care Power of Attorney forms ask the individual to make decisions related to three main end-of-life concerns. More decisions can be added, some can be eliminated, and others modified. The following are the three categories that most often appear:

- Do you want to pursue aggressive health care for a long, chronic illness?
- Do you want to be resuscitated if an illness is causing severe dementia?
- What medical treatments do you object to based on religious preferences?

As I noted earlier, each state has its own laws regarding how to draw up a Medical Care Power of Attorney. Various forms can be downloaded for free on the Internet, and if you use one, it's a good idea to have your attorney review it. A Medical Care Power of Attorney stays in effect indefinitely unless a specific termination date is given. However, it can be revoked at any time.

Do Not Resuscitate

This document specifies the conditions under which extraordinary measures to sustain life are to be avoided. It doesn't mean that non-life-threatening emergencies can't be treated. Many people believe that a DNR isn't needed when a Medical Care Power of Attorney has been filed, since a caregiver can make a critical decision concerning resuscitation when necessary. But a problem may arise when the caregiver is not available at the time of an emergency. If paramedics are called or your loved one enters a hospital and you are not present, then personnel are obligated to sustain his or her life unless a legal document says they shouldn't.

Sometimes even the existence of a DNR is not sufficient if its location is not known. The wife of one patient left for a few hours to run errands and had a relative sit with her husband. When he started having severe chest pains related to an end-stage heart condition, the relative mistakenly called paramedics instead of the hospice service. By the time the paramedics arrived, the man was unconscious. The relative said she knew he had filed a DNR, but didn't know where it was and was unable to contact his wife. The paramedics felt they had no choice but to revive him. They saved his life through chest compressions and intubation. He was resuscitated but remained in a vegetative state until his death three weeks later. To prevent future tragedies of this type, the hospice service made sure that a DNR form was conspicuously placed in the home of each patient who had filed one, and that the location of the document was known to everyone caring for a patient. Most facilities caring for elderly or ill people routinely keep DNRs close to the patient — posted on a bulletin board in the patient's room, attached to the wall above the bed, or placed in some other easy-to-find location.

A DNR gives an immediate message to all medical staff, and at a time of crisis it sends a quicker "stop" than a Medical Care Power of Attorney document. That's because, if no specific instructions are available, the heath care provider must speak with the person who has the power of attorney before life-sustaining procedures are withheld. DNRs frequently are filed along with other end-of-life documents, since they are universally understood and provide medical practitioners with legal cover in the case of end-of-life decisions made without the presence of the person who has the power of attorney.

Living Will

A Living Will is a legal document with which a person makes known his or her wishes regarding life-prolonging medical treatments. It is also called an Advance Directive, Health Care Directive, or a Physician's Directive. A Living Will informs health care providers and family about a person's desire for specific types of medical treatment in the event that he or she is unable to speak. In many ways, it overlaps with the Medical Care Power of Attorney. The requirements for the Living Will vary across states, so you'll want to have an attorney either prepare or review yours. A Living Will becomes effective only when a person can't communicate. And usually the document states that a physician must certify that your loved one is either suffering from a terminal illness or permanently unconscious before it can be implemented. A Living Will is used only when there is no hope for recovery.

Five Wishes

The Five Wishes booklet is a form of Living Will that documents how a person wants to be cared for if he or she becomes seriously ill and unable to make decisions. It addresses the following five wishes:

- Who will make health care decisions on behalf of the person named in the document.

- The kind of medical treatment he or she wants or doesn't want.
- How comfortable he or she wants to be.
- How he or she wants people to medically treat him or her.
- What he or she wants family or a significant other to know.

The booklet was written with the help of the American Bar Association's Commission on Legal Problems of the Elderly and end-of-life experts. All your loved one need do is check a box, circle a direction, or write a few sentences. Its simplicity is, ironically, both its strength and its weakness. Placing a mark on a piece of paper makes completing the form easy. But that also allows loved ones to avoid discussing some of the most important concerns they might have. I suggest discussing each wish before writing down preferences. The Five Wishes document meets the legal requirements for a Living Will in forty-two states and is useful in all fifty. It is available in twenty-six languages.

Physician Orders for Life-Sustaining Treatment

The POLST is a relatively new form that lets individuals state what kind of medical treatment they want toward the end of life. To be legal, it must be signed by both the individual and a physician. It's printed on bright pink paper, making it stand out even in a full medical folder. Some end-of-life specialists believe that this document gives seriously ill patients more control over their care than other documents because it is more specific. The decisions listed in the POLST form include whether the patient wants medical personnel to do the following:

- Attempt cardiopulmonary resuscitation
- Administer antibiotics and intravenous fluids
- Use a ventilator to help with breathing
- Provide nutrition by tube

Those who created the POLST didn't intend for it to replace the Living Will, but rather to complement it. If there is a conflict between the POLST and the Living Will, the more recent document is followed. If your loved one is incapacitated, you can sign the document if you already have the Medical Care Power of Attorney. As with any end-of-life document, you should retain the original POLST form and provide copies to the hospital or care facility, physicians, other health care providers, family members, and your attorney. You should, preferably, print the copies on pink paper, as the original is.

The POLST, just like any other end-of-life form, can be changed at any time if your loved one's preferences change. The developers of the POLST suggest reviewing the document when any of the following occur:

- Your loved one is transferred from one setting to another.
- There is a change in overall health.
- Treatment preferences change for any reason.

In the event that your loved one is transferred to a new facility without the POLST, faxed copies are valid.

Conservatorship or Guardianship

Conservatorship or guardianship should be considered the last resort in protecting the interests of a loved one. This legal procedure is most often resorted to when none of the other arrangements listed in this section have been completed and the person who needs protection is unable to make sound decisions regarding self or property. The court can be petitioned to assign a conservator or guardian when there is a dispute between family members, or when someone attempting to make decisions for the person in question is viewed as a predator and there are no legal documents available to prevent financial or physical harm. Conservatorship is appropriate when financial matters are at issue, and guardianship is appropriate when health and welfare matters are at issue.

A concerned individual or institution files a petition with the court to begin either process. During the hearing, a judge determines whether the individual has the capacity to make day-to-day decisions. If the capacity is lacking, a conservator or guardian — which can be either an individual or an institution — is appointed to take on that responsibility. This draconian method of protecting a loved one can be avoided when the forms outlined earlier in this section are completed.

WHERE TO DIE

Deciding where to die is not a macabre fixation. Decisions tend to be a consequence of one's perspective on living. Sometimes, when no options are available, the course of dying may be determined by a facility's policies and capabilities. It's never just a choice of where to die, but also of how. Talking about the different places available will give you insight into your loved one's needs.

In a Hospital

People who have decided that every medical effort should be made until their bodies give up will most likely be limited to ending life in a hospital, since few nursing homes, skilled nursing facilities, and patients' homes can be equipped with the devices and staff necessary for heroic measures. The decision to die in a hospital has the underlying premise that the length of time left to live is more important than the quality of time remaining. As noted earlier, it's a commonly held belief among the general population and many physicians that not being told you are dying can provide an extended period of life because hope for a recovery is kept alive. But the opposite was shown in an end-of-life study reported in the *Canadian Journal of Medicine* on March 14, 2010. Researchers found that people in hospices lived longer than in acute care facilities, such as hospitals. It's been my experience that patients who receive hospice services often exceed their physicians' predictions concerning how much time they have left. I believe this has much to do with a hospice facility's calmer approach to caring, its caregivers' compassion, and the reduced amount of activity in the patients' vicinity. It is much easier to think about your life and get closure in a quiet room filled with treasured pictures and memorabilia — where there are no restrictions on visits by family and friends — than when attached to intravenous lines and monitors in a sterile hospital room while attended by endless groups of interns and while listening to incessant sounds coming from the hallway.

After prostate surgery, I was placed in a room with an older man whose colon cancer had metastasized. Even though the surgeon had tried to remove the cancerous tissue, it was widespread, and little could be done. He explained this to the patient and his family while I lay on the other side of a curtain that divided the room. The corridor was filled with all the usual sounds associated with a busy hospital. The patient was clearly in the process of dying, and his relatives were trying to say their final good-byes amid the sounds of his monitors, the constant interruption of nurses, and the occasional visits by small groups of interns. Excellent though the hospital was, the requirements of caring for patients in a teaching environment trumped the needs of a family who sought the peacefulness necessary to say their final good-byes.

At Home with a Hospice Service

If a decision is made to stop curative treatments and provide only palliative care, then hospice services in your home are appropriate. But the use of a hospice service can be problematic if the patient's terminal status has been withheld. To receive hospice services, a patient and his or her physician, and sometimes a family member, must sign a document acknowledging that the patient has six months or less to live and only palliative medicines or treatment will be used. I imagine that, with a Medical Care Power of Attorney, an attempt could be made to keep secret the terminal status of a loved one, since the document could be signed by the legal designate. But while this might be a way around the issue, the potential for creating a loss of trust is substantial. If a patient is alert, the use of a Medical Care Power of Attorney may not be accepted for enrollment in hospice services.

Family members who are reluctant to tell loved ones they have a terminal condition often hold off on calling a hospice until very late in the dying process. The average use of hospice services nation-wide lasts fourteen to twenty days. But if physicians state that patients have six months or less to live, these patients can immediately qualify for services. So why the delay? Psychologically, it is difficult to acknowledge that nothing more can be done to save someone's life. But by not telling a loved one she is dying, compassionate, comprehensive care may be needlessly delayed.

There is comfort in preparing to die in your own home, in the bed you have rested in for years, surrounded by what's most meaningful to you. I had one patient who was living in an apartment in a run-down area of San Francisco, whose entire living space consisted of a small room with a shared bathroom down the hallway. When he could no longer care for himself, and the chaotic and unsanitary condition of the apartment made it impossible for health care workers to provide the services he needed, he was placed in a stand-alone hospice. His room, though small, was clean and cheery and was served by caring staff twenty-four hours a day. When I met him, he said, "You know, this place is very nice, but it's not my home." For him, the squalor of his one-room apartment was familiar. That's where he wanted to die. If your loved one is reluctant to move to a facility, understand that this is a common reaction. It's not your commitment that is being questioned. As with many aspects of end-of-life issues, it's not about you.

In a Stand-Alone Care Facility or Hospice

A stand-alone hospice or other care facility may be necessary if the physical needs of your loved one exceed what you or home health care workers are able to provide. Care in such facilities is around the clock. The setting may be ideal for both patient and caregiver. When all of a loved one's physical needs are met, caregivers can focus on emotional needs.

But as noted, placement in a stand-alone hospice facility is often delayed. Be aware, too, that in most locales either the number of people needing beds in hospices exceeds the beds available, or the care is too expensive if not covered by their insurance or Medicare. For these reasons, if a stand-alone hospice facility or a nursing care facility is a possibility, it makes sense to begin your search early in order to budget your finances and place your loved one on a waiting list. Also, the early introduction of the hospice concept provides a loved one with more time to accept the idea.

One patient said to me that, until he signed the admission papers for a hospice service, he didn't believe he was dying. "Seeing those words *less than six months* made it real. And if it didn't, signing my name, saying I understood what it meant, brought it home." That was the first time he realized he was dying despite the fact that his brother had been told about it by the physician three months earlier. That information could have been used to begin discussing his imminent death. At a workshop I gave, a participant said he was reluctant to place his mother in hospice because it would signal that he had "given up" on her. When he finally began talking about hospice, it was almost four months after the terminal prognosis. Instead of gradually introducing her to the idea of hospice, it was presented at the time of her greatest anxiety and vulnerability: only weeks before her death.

OTHER HARD DECISIONS

One caregiver said to me, "The hard decisions never stop coming. Just when I think I'm through with them, up pops another." In caregiving, everything continually changes, and difficult decisions should be made as early as possible, before changes become nonstop.

Last Wishes Notebook

Janice lived alone and, except for help she received from an agency caregiver who came to her home for two hours a day, took care of her basic needs herself. The first time I visited her, she told me to sit on a couch while she went to retrieve something for me to look at.

"Here," she said, sitting down next to me and opening a folder covered with pictures of flowers and quotes from religious figures. "This is my 'I'm going to kick the bucket' book." In it were tabbed sections with the headings "How I Die," "Favorite Foods and Drinks," "Places," "People," "Things to Do," and "Places to See." Under these headings, Janice had listed things like how she wanted to die, what she wanted to do before she died, what should be done at her memorial service, and what should be done after she died. The first tab marked the place of legal forms her attorney and accountant had helped her complete. In the "Places to See" section, some of the items were checked, and she had written comments describing what she felt while experiencing them. That first time I visited, and on subsequent visits, she brought out the book and we talked about what she had accomplished during the week and what still needed doing. The conversations were about more than just going through checklists. Each became a story about something important in her life. "You know," Janice said at one visit, "I thought going to the

Napa vineyards would be something I would miss. But it can't compare with just sitting quietly in my backyard."

It was the first time I had seen such a notebook or even thought about it. And it was a rock of stability when the chaos in Janice's life became overwhelming. You may want to help your loved one construct one of these. There can be tabbed sections for forms, activities to be done, places to visit, who gets what, favorite foods, financial and legal documents (other than end-of-life documents, which should have their own tabbed section at the beginning of the notebook), questions for health care providers, and whatever else will make transitions easier. This is not something to be done at one sitting. Rather, as topics come up, memorialize them in the notebook. The time to begin is right after the prognosis.

It will become easy, as an illness progresses, to forget what was thought to be important last month, last week, or even yesterday. Relying on memory, especially during this time, can be difficult. A simple binder with tabs for different sections can relieve much of the burden on a loved one's memory, just as it did for Janice. It became a book of life rather than a morbid collection of things to do before dying.

Creating a Memorial Service

Some people insist on writing their own obituaries and on setting the conditions for their memorial services. Although it may be thought a bit too controlling, being involved in creating a memorial service long before it's needed can enable loved ones to put their lives into perspective and feel they are reducing the grief of those they leave behind. I listened to one man tell his wife that he knew how upset his grandson would be after his death. That, more than anything else, bothered him. His wife agreed that the boy would be devastated. Together, this man and his wife spent time crafting a final missive for the grandson that would be read at the memorial service. It spoke about how important the grandson was in the man's life and how, through the good deeds of the grandson, the memory of his grandfather would live.

Final Resting Place

Many people have thought about this, but few talk about it. And it's usually approached with great solemnity. But it doesn't have to be. With humor, it can become a gateway for exploring issues that have nothing to do with the final disposition of the body. One client who was seeing me for a problem when I was still a speech-language pathologist had had his leg amputated because of diabetes. He explained to me that, as he was an Orthodox Jew, tradition dictated that his leg should be buried with the remainder of his body. "Well," he said during one of our sessions, "I now have one foot in the grave." After we both laughed, he became more serious. "You know, I don't know how much time I have left."

His concern was legitimate because the severity of his diabetes was rapidly increasing. For Frank, the use of humor made a difficult topic more accessible. It can also lead in other positive directions, as it did with my wife and me. We have a favorite hike in the Carmel Valley of California that gives us joy for different reasons. There's a spot halfway through the hike where I stop and play my Native American flute or my *shakuhachi*. My wife, not a fan of either instrument, usually continues walking to a stretch on this ridge trail where she can look at a distant mountain range. But on one occasion, she stood nearby as I played.

"When I die," I said to her after I finished, "I want some of my ashes spread here."

"Why?" she said.

"Because there are few places where I feel more connected with my music than on this spot."

"Well, I don't want my ashes spread here, I want them down

there," she said, pointing to the spot about a quarter of a mile away where she would stop to look across the valley at the mountain range while I played.

"All right," I said. "We'll have the kids lay a line of ashes so we're still connected."

As we walked down the trail, we talked about how each would memorialize the other's life, what friends we would want to share the event with, and how we would relate this bizarre story to our grown children. Whether it's the disposition of a body or any of the other practical and important decisions that need to be made, I've found that dealing with an issue of this type is like pulling a loose piece of yarn from a knitted blanket — it just keeps unwinding. And in the case of my wife and me that day, issues important to how we would remember each other came up for the first time.

FINAL THOUGHTS

Life is analogous to a complicated piece of music, such as Mahler's Fifth Symphony or Billy Strayhorn's "Take the A Train." In both you can hear numerous instruments, the chord changes, the variations, and so on. But if you really want to understand the piece, you reduce it down to its basic melody. From there everything else develops. When someone is learning to accept a chronic illness or is dying, it's the melody of her life that she strives to hear and wants others to experience. She is struggling to find a place in a world that has cruelly stripped her of many things that gave her pleasure.

Where understanding is possible, we can learn how loved ones wish to be treated and what they fear. When we know these things, words and behaviors that may seem inexplicable will become more acceptable. But as the illness progresses, there may be words and behaviors so hurtful that we take them as a direct attack on us. They rarely are. When you feel most vulnerable to a loved one's accusations, that's when you need to accept that it is the illness speaking and not the loved one who, over the years, has shown you great kindness. The basic melody of her life is still there; you just need to listen more carefully to hear it.

As your loved one struggles to adapt to a world that's changing, and not necessarily for the better, she may choose less-than-skillful ways of expressing her needs. When possible, focus on what's still good and enjoyable in her life; and when you cannot, then accept what isn't. The melody of her life remains, even though what surrounds it may be discordant. If your expectations of appreciation or gratitude go unfulfilled, it won't be because you aren't doing what you should, or because your loved one doesn't understand the effort you're making. She will be struggling with some of the most difficult psychological issues there are and may be simultaneously seeing the world through pain.

Although spirituality is important for finding peace before death, it may be more important to tie up loose ends that may have haunted your loved one for her entire life. As the world she knew prior to her illness dissolves, she will look to restructure it. It most cases, that won't be possible, but you can help her find alternatives. These won't replace what she has lost, but they will partially fill the increasing number of potholes that are developing. You can do simple things to help, such as physically constructing an environment in which the artifacts of life are emphasized and those of illness are minimized.

Your loved one may become someone she doesn't want to be but has no choice but to be. Her identity will change, and so should your expectations about what she should feel and do. Losing abilities is devastating. Allow your loved one to set the pace of her growing dependence once she has accepted who she is becoming. Not all changes will be negative, but none should be glorified as a "good" outcome of the illness.

When her bodily systems break down, your loved one will need to adapt to this. You can help by simplifying her life. It can be as easy as reducing noise; or it can be more difficult, as when she must give up lifelong activities. When people's chronic and terminal illnesses spiral out of control, they abandon their emotional defense mechanisms. There is too little time left for them to pretend something exists when it doesn't or to try to present an impervious exterior that will not help them come to terms with what is happening to them.

While the changes in your loved one's body and mind are occurring, she will still be forced to function in a world that, while physically the same as her pre-illness one, has changed emotionally. Stability and predictability will be elusive. For example, the home that was a comfortable dwelling becomes a prison. The noises that gave life to the neighborhood become impediments to thinking. The world you have shared becomes irreparably changed. And although many bridges will still connect the two of you, you will need to be sensitive to the fact that your loved one's world is now different.

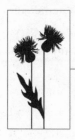

CHAPTER 4

Conversations
Words and Other Things

*I*f someone asked you, "What is a conversation?" you would probably think about the back-and-forth verbal interaction between
two or more people. You say something, then someone else says
something, and then it's your turn again. But conversations are significantly more than that. Hidden beneath the words may be specific
intentions that can lead to unforeseen reactions. For example, how
do you feel when someone doesn't respond to something important
you said, but goes off on an unrelated topic, leaving you hanging
there with an unfinished discussion? Or how often have you wanted
to have a back-and-forth conversation with someone but were put in
the position of continually responding to questions?

Conversations can range from the highly directed question-and-
answer type found between teachers and students in an elementary
school to the open-ended questions found in psychotherapy sessions.
The outcomes of conversations between you and your loved one
may be determined more by their structure than by your intentions.

THE CONTENT

This is the "meat" of a message. The content may appear to be just
information, but in fact, there may be hidden layers that affect how

loved ones interpret it. Very rarely is the content of messages between caregivers and loved ones simple information. Whether intended or not, emotions are often embedded in our words, in ways we may not be aware of. And sometimes the messages of loved ones are communicated in bizarre ways.

One of my Alzheimer's patients was moved from his apartment to the skilled nursing care wing of an assisted living facility. When I arrived, he was repetitively rubbing his finger on the blanket. One of his attendants said he had been doing that for four days, but nobody could understand what it meant. According to the attendant: "It's just one of those Alzheimer's things patients do." I noticed that the blanket had been tightly tucked under his feet. I pulled the blanket from under his feet, releasing the tension, and the repetitive motion stopped. Always look for the communicative intent of behaviors, even though words aren't being used.

Clarifying What We Say

We often think of our words as simply symbols conveying factual information. We have something to say, and we think it doesn't make much difference which words we choose to express it as long as the information is accurately presented. For example, when you need to go to the store, you say to your loved one, "I need to go to the store." Or, when you're exhausted, you say, "I'm going to sleep for an hour." In both cases you're expressing your needs. There's nothing wrong with that. But how would your message be interpreted if you rephrased these sentences in the following way: "I need to go to the store; *will you be all right here alone for thirty minutes?*" "I'm exhausted and I need to sleep for an hour. *Is there anything I can do for you before I lie down?*" While both the original sentences and the revisions convey the same information, the second set shows sensitivity to your loved one's needs. And that sensitivity often has important consequences.

Recently, I served a woman in her eighties. I visited her twice in an extended care facility, and on my third visit I met her daughter. It was important that I convey some information to her daughter, and she felt the same need to give me an update on the condition of her mother, who had had a stroke three days before my visit. Before we began speaking, she said, "Mom, Stan and I need to talk about you. We know you can hear and understand everything we will be saying, but for the time being, we won't be including you in the conversation. Is that all right?" The reaction of her mother was positive. The daughter could have just as easily said, "Mom, Stan and I need to talk about you now," or even not said anything to her about the conversation. Sometimes, just the addition of a few words that acknowledge your loved one's needs can do much to convey your compassion, even when you believe your message is just informational.

When Things Become Frightening

By waiting until your loved one is ready to talk about something frightening, there's a greater probability that he will be able to discuss it with less fear. That was the case with Mary and Joe. Joe had been told in his doctor's office that his congestive heart failure would result in his death within a few months. Stoically, he accepted the news as if he had been told he had some minor condition. But when they got home, his wife said later, he held her hand and cried. "I know this is very frightening for you," Mary told him. "I'm scared, too. I just want you to know that when you're ready to talk, I'll be here to listen." She sat next to him and bore witness to his emotional pain. The next day, he carried on as if the terminal diagnosis had been just a figment of his imagination. He talked about a trip he wanted to take with her to Africa the following year and a remodeling project he was planning. Although she knew neither would happen, she didn't confront him. In conversations with me, she said she felt he wasn't ready to talk about his death, and until he was, she would wait. Three weeks later Joe was admitted into hospice service after his congestive heart failure resulted in edema (water retention) throughout his body.

"I never believed the docs knew what they were talking about," he said. "I knew I was going to die, but maybe in five years. I agreed to hospice care because I knew that would make Mary feel better. But now, my body is telling me it's going to fail soon."

"Do you want to talk to Mary about it?" I asked.

"Yes, but if I do, she'll know I'm dying."

The previous week Mary had taken me aside when her husband was sleeping and said, "I know he's dying, but I'm afraid to say anything about it. I'm sure he still thinks he has a lot of time left." When I was alone with Joe, I said, "I think it will be all right for you to talk about these things with Mary." When I returned the following week, Joe told me they had started talking about his death when I left, and continued the conversation each day.

Mary could have persisted in wanting to talk about Joe's impending death when he was denying that it would soon occur, but she didn't. We often try to make loved ones "face reality," whether it involves the acceptance of a chronic illness or their impending death. But, as I wrote earlier, the reality of a healthy person is different from the reality of someone with a progressive illness. A caregiver's idea of when it's time to talk about important issues may be different from that of her loved one.

When the Words Mean Something Else

A caregiver may look at a loved one's problems and try to address the specifics. Your loved one isn't eating properly, so you talk about nutrition. He isn't quite as diligent as is necessary about his medication, so you explain why it's important to take pills routinely. He is ignoring the advice of the nurse and moving around more than he should, so you explain why he must remain less active. Each problem is specific and potentially life threatening. So you do what you should as a caregiver: you try to keep him on track. And when he ignores your perfectly logical suggestions, you may think he's being "difficult" or drifting into dementia. While both explanations are possible, often the problem goes beyond the specifics, especially when loved ones acknowledge that they know what they should be doing but aren't doing it.

When your loved one's decisions don't make sense — whatever the reason — it may be time to explore some of the larger issues, like his acceptance of what is happening to him or the knowledge that he may be on a fast track to death. One elderly mother refused to eat or drink, and her daughter's initial interpretation was that this was her mother's way of getting attention from other family members. The daughter's response was to get angry with her mother for being manipulative. In a subsequent conversation that the mother had with her own sister, she was very clear that it was time to die, and not eating was a conscious decision she had made to hasten her death. She wasn't trying to manipulate anyone. I believe it usually makes sense to give loved ones the benefit of the doubt, to assume that their decisions are logical, even though they may appear bizarre.

Actions Rather Than Words

Throughout caregiving, you will constantly be given the chance to express love and compassion. Never miss the opportunity to use the words, but don't assume that the words are substitutes for actions. Forget about large gestures; think of something small, immediate, and meaningful. When I was serving a very proper retired university professor, I noticed his urinal was full and it appeared that he needed to use it. Without saying anything, I took it to the bathroom and emptied it. I replaced it on his wheelchair and said, "I'll be back in a few minutes." When I returned, he thanked me profusely. It was a small act I performed, but one that enabled him to hold on to his dignity; and until he died, that one act was something for which he continually thanked me. A loved one's perception of a caregiver's compassion is related to the little things that have immediate consequences. Aspiring writers composing fiction are often told: "Show, don't tell." In caregiving, a similarly useful maxim is: Intentionally show your compassion; don't merely spend time telling your loved one how much you care.

THE DYNAMICS OF CONVERSATIONS

There is an ebb and flow to conversations that may appear seamless, but isn't. Attending to what is said is more complicated than most of us realize. We assume loved ones need only listen or watch. But what does listening and watching require? One often hears the story — true or not — that a butterfly flapping its wings in Africa can, eventually, start a hurricane in the Atlantic Ocean. Conversations have the same dynamics. Their structure continually changes according to what is said and what each person brings to the table.

When I was still counseling, I was always aware of the sequence of my interactions with clients. Before saying something, I would anticipate what they would say and how I would respond, and then how they would respond to my response. The experience made it evident to me just how dynamic conversations are and what could enhance and impede them. Many simple things, ranging from just listening rather than talking, to the tone of a conversation, can determine how positive an outcome will be.

Listen More, Talk Less

In our normal lives, we often seek to fill silence with words. I've found this to be especially true in the presence of someone who is dying. Many believe that as people approach death, their need to communicate diminishes. Actually, the reverse is true. Unfortunately, we misperceive a reduction in words as a reduction in need. People who are dying are facing the most profound transition they've ever encountered. Everything about them is changing. Silence is not necessarily a sign of not wishing to communicate or wishing visitors would fill the void. It may signal great uncertainty or fear. Dying people want to communicate, but within their own time frames.

At a workshop on death and dying, the noted Tibetan Buddhist monk Sogyal Rinpoche said that lectures were for entertainment, silence for deep learning. I think that can equally be applied to how caregivers interact with loved ones. We are used to filling silence with words because of our discomfort, and these filler conversations often have little substance. Take the following dialogue I listened to when relatives visited one of my patients.

"Ari, you're looking so much better," his cousin said. Ari knew that he wasn't looking better. As his HIV progressed, the hollows of his eyes became deeper and his shirt draped over his body as if he were a child trying on his father's clothes. When he didn't say anything, the cousin continued.

"Well, you know, it's such a lovely day today, maybe we can go out on the deck?" After fifteen seconds elapsed and Ari still hadn't said anything, she said, "Would you like to see some pictures of the trip we made to Tahoe?"

She wasn't being insensitive. But like many people, she believed that silence was meant to be filled. I wondered whether this final interaction between my patient and his cousin would have been different had she remained quiet until Ari was ready to speak. And how would the conversation have affected the last week of his life and his cousin's memories of him if Ari had been given the time to compose his thoughts? Before talking to loved ones during those uncomfortable silent periods, ask yourself if the words you are about to say are necessary or just meant to fill an uncomfortable gap. It's rarely an issue of a loved one feeling uncomfortable with the silence. Silence may be necessary for preparing to share difficult thoughts with you. Can you convey what you feel just by your presence or a touch, or by simply holding your loved one's hand?

What would happen if you remained silent? Silence allows space for loved ones to begin difficult conversations. This is when the past and a limited future run wild in their minds, as I think happened for a client who was described in his chart as a paranoid schizophrenic. He refused to talk to anyone during the first three days at his new facility. "Hi, I'm Stan," I said as I sat down next to his bed. He had advanced lung cancer and wasn't expected to live for more than a month. "I'm a volunteer from Pathways." I waited for him to respond. He nodded and turned his head toward the wall on the other side of his bed. I sat in the chair and calmly looked across the room. Almost one hour elapsed without either of us speaking. I stood, preparing to leave, and was about to ask him if he would like me to return the following week.

"I'm afraid of dying," he said.

I sat back down. He turned his head away from me and stared at the wall again. Ten minutes later he turned toward me. "What's it like?" he asked.

He was able to voice his fears, not because of any counseling skills that I possessed, but because I had the sense to keep my mouth shut. It began the pattern of our interactions until he died three weeks later. I would say something and wait for his response. Sometimes it was immediate; at other times it could take five or ten minutes for him to become comfortable enough to talk. Occasionally, he would have me put together an old Lionel model train set on the floor, and I would run it until he felt comfortable talking. What loved ones may want to talk about may not be as dramatic as the concerns of my patient, but giving someone the space to talk often gives them permission to deal with difficult topics. It takes more time to prepare for talking about the big issues, such as the need to be forgiven, than for discussing how the Giants are doing in the pennant race.

Reduce Noise

When we think about noise, we usually have a constricted view of it. To someone who has lived in rural areas, the hum of a car's tires on a smooth road might be considered noise. To an urban dweller visiting the country, it's the crickets that produce an unbearable racket. Basically, noise is anything that interferes with receiving or delivering a message, or that disrupts a loved one's mental state. For an ill person, it could be a vacuum cleaner in the apartment next door, a television incessantly delivering unwanted messages, or even the babble created when two or more people are trying to talk at the same time. The more noise that is present, the harder becomes the work of dealing with chronic and terminal illnesses.

I served a woman in a nursing home whose staff was overworked. When I visited, the television at the foot of her bed was constantly on, at a volume I found excessive. Stepping out into the hallway, I could hear other televisions blaring, many tuned to different stations. The cacophony of sounds reminded me of an airport with simultaneous announcements. The explanation from one staff member was that television served as a "distraction." It did, but it was a distraction from preparing to die. Noise can be neutral in terms of intention (it's just there) or used as a way of minimizing the impact or discomfort of a person's distress. But as long as the television was blaring, staff couldn't hear patients, nor could a patient call to staff after the call button was pressed. Don't assume your loved one wants to be distracted. Always ask if it's all right before turning on a television, radio, or CD player. And when having a conversation, turn off all media.

In our daily lives, we often use noise as a way to isolate us from our surroundings. Yes, the proliferation of earbuds plugged into iPods may indicate a growing appreciation of music, but I suspect it has more to do with a desire to insulate ourselves from the world. For loved ones with progressive illnesses, noise, whether it is street traffic or a reality show on television, interferes with the final sorting out of thoughts.

Your loved one needs to pull important messages out of the sur-rounding noise. For most people, it's not a problem. We seem to use some type of filter that allows the important messages to get through while suppressing ones that aren't. For example, the television is on and someone starts speaking to you from the next room. Although the sound of the television is louder than that person's voice, you can still attend to the message coming from the kitchen. However, as a loved one's thinking is compromised by illness, her neurological filter, which separates noise from important messages, may be dif-ficult to access. We can't tell beforehand the level of noise that will affect your loved one's ability to attend to your words or her own thoughts. Regardless of the level, your goal is to decrease noise in order to accommodate her ability, which may continually be declin-ing. That may involve keeping the television or radio off when she is speaking, making sure only one person speaks at a time, or keeping things quiet when she is resting.

Who Goes First?

What I've found in listening to conversations is that the flow often depends on who starts it. In counseling, I never began sessions with what was on my agenda. It was usually: "How has the week been going for you?" When I started volunteering in hospice, I found the same approach was useful when I came for my weekly visits. An open-ended question of this type says, "I'm interested in you. Please tell me what you think is important and what you want to talk about." It often led to poignant conversations about life and death.

But sometimes a little coaxing is in order. For example, a loved one appears melancholy in the afternoon, but was jovial in the morning. A caregiver can be direct and set the agenda by saying, "You look like you're in pain; should I increase the amount of oxygen?" Or he can take a more open-ended approach by saying: "You look unhappy. Is there anything you want me to do or to talk about?" The response to either question might be the same: "Yes, turn up the oxygen." But the second question allows a loved one to talk about what's most important to her, something that may have nothing to do with the oxygen.

When and How to Begin an End-of-Life Discussion

In the 1930s there was a misguided notion in my profession — speech-language pathology — that if we used the word *stutterer* with a child, he would be traumatized. It was ludicrous to believe that a child who was teased by other children for repeating sounds and blocking on words wouldn't know he was doing something very different from other children unless the label was used. The logic used in the 1930s made as little sense as the fears people currently have in using the "D word" with loved ones who are dying. And when patients corner physicians for an answer regarding how long they have to live, even some of the most brilliant physicians stumble as if they were on a first date.

If a loved one wants to talk about dying, don't change the subject or insist that "everything will be all right." A statement such as "I think I'm dying" comes from a profound realization or fear that something very unusual is happening within a person's body or mind. Seize the opportunity to begin the discussion, as painful as it may be for both of you. It may be the first step in preparing for the end of life. Don't use euphemisms for dying unless your loved one uses them first. However, there is no reason to continually repeat *dying* and *death* throughout your conversations.

A patient diagnosed with liver cancer knew his prognosis was uncertain. His fears increased when the surgeon told him the cancer cells had metastasized. "I did what many people do after receiving terrible news," he said. "I shut down. I told my wife I was fine whenever she asked how I was doing. She told me that she would be there for me when I was ready to talk. I kept telling her I was fine." He paused and sighed deeply. "I wasn't fine then, or at any of the other times she asked during the next few months. I was so frightened by the thought of dying that I pretended I was comfortable with the possibility. Eventually, I was able to talk to her and my children about it."

In eight years of hospice volunteering I have never initiated a discussion of dying with my patients. Yet at least 80 percent of them talked about it — not when I decided it was appropriate, but when they made the decision to do so. I've found that accepting the possibility of one's death in the very near future usually precedes discussions about it. When caregivers try to force the discussion — sometimes for legitimate reasons — loved ones may become defensive. Knowing intellectually that you are facing death is not the same as accepting it in your heart, as was the case with my patient who had liver cancer.

The discussions my patient had with his wife were uncomfortable, but these became an entryway for dealing with the important issues that are usually put off until it's too late — issues such as forgiving, asking for forgiveness, expressing love, and conveying gratitude, among other things. If loved ones have always been reluctant to discuss feelings, don't expect that to change, at least not initially. I think it's important to allow them to bring up those issues when they are ready. I've found that, regardless of the phase of illness a person is experiencing, people who aren't ready to talk about dying don't. My patient became annoyed at his wife every time she wanted to talk about his health, even though he knew she was only trying to help. When he was ready, he welcomed and cherished the conversations.

When loved ones are ready, they'll talk. That doesn't mean you should ignore your own legitimate feelings of impending loss. A husband who had difficulty socializing when his wife wasn't present became terrified thinking about facing life without her. Both knew that her metastatic breast cancer would end her life within a few months. Although she accepted her fate, in the past she had never felt comfortable discussing her feelings, even with her husband. His being honest with her about how much he would miss her gave her permission to share with him her own feelings about dying. As I wrote earlier, dying is a community event, and therefore caregivers should feel they have a right to express how they feel about a loved one's condition.

Stay the Course

Imagine settling into a nice comfortable chair. The cushions mold to your body, and maybe for the first time all day you feel relaxed. Then, just as you begin to luxuriate in the feeling, someone says you'll have to move. "But I'm comfortable right here," you plead. He's not concerned; he wants you to move, *right now*. You do, but with much resentment. Your loved one may feel the same way if you try to move from one topic to another before she feels closure. Life, with its frenetic pace, seems to place little value on staying with a topic for long.

The most important news segments on television may take six minutes. A new form of fiction called flash fiction limits the telling of a story to a few pages, and sometimes even to a paragraph. Twitter allows the sender only 140 characters to disseminate a message. It's no wonder, then, that rarely do we exhaust a topic. We have a tendency to move on, believing that the more we can cram into a short amount of time, the better the interaction. The opposite is actually true — especially when we are conversing with people who have progressive illnesses. Knowing they may not have much time left, they are selective about their choice of topics. What they want to discuss rarely is of the same superficial quality as small talk.

One patient wanted to talk about why an attendant was perpetually late in giving her a bath. "You know," she said, "if she'd just call and say she'd be late, that would be fine. But she never does." My patient was in an excellent assisted living facility with very compassionate staff, and it wasn't as if she would be missing an appointment because of the lateness of the personal assistant. A typical response to her complaint would have been to agree that it was an inconsiderate thing to do, and to move on to another conversation. But I realized that her annoyance didn't make sense unless it was an indication that she had a deeper concern, especially when she kept reiterating the problem. So instead of introducing another topic, we talked about what being late meant to her. She was beginning to experience mild dementia along with the chronic heart failure that would eventually end her life. Given her feeling that she was losing stability in her life — a common feeling in dementia patients — it was important for her to cling to structure. The uncertainty of when she would be bathed interfered with that. I couldn't have known beforehand her feelings about why she was so upset with the attendant. But I was able to find out by just staying with the topic, something you can easily do with your loved one.

One very important technique that allows for probing the depths of a topic is called follow-up. When your loved one starts a conversation, you keep following up on every one of his responses. Here's an example of a conversation I had with a patient concerning a vision of his wife.

"You know, I saw her yesterday," he said.

"Who was that?"

"My wife."

"I didn't know she was still alive."

"She isn't. She died three years ago."

"That must have been a strange experience for you."

"No, it really wasn't. It was my wife. I was wide awake when I saw her at the foot of my bed. You probably think I'm nuts or just delusional."

"No, I don't. Seeing someone who is no longer alive is something many of my patients have described to me."

If you look at our interaction, you'll see that whenever I responded to my patient, I always referred to what he had just said. It will become evident to you when the topic becomes exhausted — your loved one will probably change the subject.

Don't Fight Emotional Distress

Feeling physically and emotionally lousy affects everything we do. We have trouble interacting with others. We can't concentrate. We don't operate as efficiently as we'd like. Our loved ones have similar problems, but often the breaks between feeling good and feeling lousy fluctuate wildly, or the periods of "lousy" dominate. I think the swings become more understandable when we view them as reactions to shock. Most people think of shock as having a single point of occurrence. I believe for someone who hasn't adjusted to her illness, there are multiple points. Just when she thinks she has settled into an adjustment, the illness progresses and a new shock point is initiated.

When I'm with someone who is in shock, I just listen. In 2010, there was a huge gas explosion in San Bruno, a small town just south of San Francisco. My wife was asked to register evacuees at one of the Red Cross shelters. I accompanied her and, along with other volunteers, registered those who had been evacuated or lost their homes. What became immediately evident was that most people who came into the shelter had that blank look associated with being in shock, and they wanted to talk. Many had run to safety after they watched homes on their block ignite. Interviewers who rigidly held to a script for getting information got only the information they sought. But those of us who listened, and allowed the periods of silence to be filled by what the evacuees wanted to say, heard them describe traumatic events and express terrifying emotions. For many, it was the first time they had spoken about their experiences. Even though we allowed them to talk as much as they wanted, we eventually got the information requested by the Red Cross.

Shock is not always confined to a specific event. Some loved ones who seem to have adjusted to their situation may be, without any warning, overcome with the realization of what is or will be happening to them. It is during those times that you should allow the silence to continue until your loved one is ready to discuss what she is feeling. Sometimes the most important information about her feelings will be expressed during those periods of silence when you may be struggling to think of what you can do to fill them.

Go Slowly

We often talk to our loved ones as if they can process information with the same ease that they did before becoming ill. But people's ability to process information can be affected by pain, medication, or difficulty in accepting their new and ever-changing status. The simple act of slowing down your speech can ease the difficulty. I dread having to call a customer service department when I know that at the other end of the line will be someone with a foreign accent. It's nothing cultural. Rather, as someone with a hearing impairment, I know I will miss much of what is said, and the electronic device I'm calling about will remain unfixed. Most of the representatives who handle customer service that has been outsourced to other countries not only speak English with a pronounced accent but also speak at rates in excess of two hundred words per minute. Not a great situation for an older person with a hearing problem.

One would think that, as a speech-language pathologist, I would be more adept at pulling out meaning even when the accents are difficult to understand. Generally that was true before my hearing began to deteriorate. Now, with my need to concentrate on just hearing the message, I often have to ask the representative to repeat or slow down. Since it's difficult for others to constantly monitor their rate of speech, what little relief I'm given by a reduced rate is lost after about fifteen seconds, when the speaker's rate soars back to more than two hundred words per minute.

Loved ones with normal hearing may have similar experiences. While my difficulty in attending to the content of the message is related to a hearing impairment, your loved one's difficulty in listening to you may come from physical or psychological pain. Whenever I'm with patients, I try to slow down. They may not need me to do that, but I never know what issues they are dealing with. Slowing your speech rate is an easy and nonintrusive way of helping your loved one understand what you are saying. Reducing your rate to below one hundred words per minute has a great effect on understanding. You don't have to make any complicated measurements. Just think about speaking slower, regardless of the rate you are using, as long as it sounds normal. If you want to be more precise, record yourself for five minutes and divide the total number of words you spoke by five.

One Phrase, One Idea

How often have you gone to a presentation on a topic you really wanted to learn more about and heard the presenter linking endless ideas together? A sentence would go on and on, becoming a paragraph of up to one hundred words, and, remarkably, the speaker would never stop to take a breath! You really tried to understand all the ideas, but if you took more than a millisecond to digest one, you'd miss the next three. The normal processing of information is more complicated than most people understand. If speakers truly understood that fact, then, for example, the salesman trying to sell you an item would present you with only one idea, or only a few ideas, to process before inserting a break into his message.

The more stress a loved one is experiencing, the more time is needed to process incoming information. I mentioned the importance of slowing down your speech rate. Introducing pauses between ideas is a complementary strategy. When two or more ideas are contained in a sentence, the possibility of losing one is increased. Pause between ideas. The more ideas presented without an opportunity to process them, the more likely they will be forgotten or misinterpreted. For example, here are two different ways of presenting the same ideas. Read each example out loud and choose which style you would want to listen to. Which style would allow you to retain the most information if the presentation lasted thirty minutes?

Example 1

- In order to make this oxygen-generating machine function effectively, all of the knobs on the top of the panel, especially those that are green, need to be set to zero before the valve at the top next to the main line is activated and the line is released.

Example 2

- Find the knobs on top of the panel.
- Make sure that all knobs are set to zero.
- Activate the main line by releasing it.

Our minds have the capacity to turn themselves off when the information given to us exceeds our capacity to process it. Instead of listening, we dream, focus on a person sitting in front of us, maybe even decide what we will cook for dinner. Anything other than torturing our overtired minds with endless ideas that flow into each other as if they were tributaries rushing into a large river.

Choosing Words and Sentence Structure

I become easily confused when I have to choose between different types of electronic equipment. When I decided to substitute a digital camera for my old thirty-five-millimeter Nikon, I asked the salesperson for a "PhD" camera. He looked confused and said, "I'm sorry, sir, we only have Nikons, Fujis, and Canons. We don't carry the PhD brand." My attempt at being humorous failed. "No," I said. "A PhD camera is a 'Push here, dummy' one. You know, the type that's so simple it requires me only to push one button." He smiled. "Oh, yes, sir, we have many models for people like you."

With some chronic and terminal illnesses, simplifying messages can help, and with all forms of dementia it's important. You can make the message more understandable by using less complex words and simpler grammar. I had a patient who grew up in Oklahoma during the Depression. His family lived on a small farm, and his father kept him out of school so he could work the fields. Although he never went to school, he taught himself to read. While his speech often expressed sophisticated ideas, he didn't have the five-dollar words to deliver them.

"You know," he said, "I only feel comfortable talking to you and the nurse."

"Why?" I said.

"Both of you use words I understand. Some of the other people who come to the house use words I never heard."

"Do you ask them what they mean?"

"No, I never do. If I did that, they would know I never had any schooling. And then what would they think about me?"

For my patient, it was important to present an image of someone who could be respected. To preserve that image, he was willing to listen to important information he didn't understand without questioning it. And since his wife had had a stroke a number of years before he started receiving hospice services, there wasn't anyone in the home who would understand how important the information was. As a result, financial help that was available to him for paying utilities, for example, was never accessed.

Choosing a simpler way to communicate doesn't mean that your loved one has lost the ability to understand complexities. Rather, the changes in body and brain are making it more difficult to process information. It's as if your loved one's brain is running at twenty miles per hour and the world is going by at eighty. The car's engine still works, but just a little slower. Match the speed and use twenty-five-cent words rather than five-dollar ones, and many of the processing problems will be reduced or eliminated.

The Tone of Conversations

Many years ago, when my daughter was in her teens, we would have conversations about our conversations. "It's not what you say, Daddy, it's how you say it." What she was able to pick up from my speech was that, even though I thought my words were unambiguous and neutral when I gave her directions on what to do with her life, my feelings were often conveyed by my tone. What researchers found in much of the early analysis of nonverbal behaviors in the 1970s was that often the intent of a message was discerned by how it was said. We all seem to have a built-in "truth meter" that compares the words in someone's speech with the way he says it. When those things are in agreement, we say to ourselves, "Yes, I understand what this person is saying and feeling." But when the words say one thing and the tone another, we go to the tone to find the feeling behind the words, or what we think the person really means.

There will be times when you may not be as compassionate as you would like, as patient as you want to be, or as understanding as your loved one needs you to be. At times like these and other distressful ones, you may try to convey your ideal self to your loved one with the words you choose. We are more aware of our words than our tone. And our inability to monitor tone can make it easier for loved ones to identify what we are feeling, regardless of what the words mean. Some people choose to rigorously monitor both their words and their tone to convey a unified message to loved ones. That's often true of those who fear expressing their true feelings. You may find you are momentarily successful with this approach, but continually monitoring tone takes an enormous amount of effort, and, just as my daughter did, your loved one will probably pick up on the discrepancy. The solution? Don't be afraid to express your emotions, since most likely your loved one will detect them anyway.

OTHER WAYS OF COMMUNICATING

As a practicing speech-language pathologist for more than thirty years, I worked to help people become more proficient in the use of language. I believed that communicating what was true and important was best done with words. My first hospice patient taught me the folly of my thinking. Of course words are important for conveying information. But there are emotions that words are inadequate to communicate. Think about the most beautiful sunset you ever witnessed. When you saw your first newborn child. For musicians, that piece you played that you thought came from the heavens. For athletes, the movement you couldn't believe your body executed. For writers, an incredible paragraph you just typed and wondered who wrote it. And for most people, the moment you realized you had found your soul mate.

There are no words for these types of experiences and for many of the feelings you may wish to convey to your loved one. But you can express them through what I call "heart communications." These are nonverbal expressions of emotions, such as holding a loved one's hand, that contain a minimum of analytical rigor and a maximum of unadorned honesty. Start using heart communications early in chronic and terminal illnesses, so when your loved one can no longer use or understand words, a comfortable and familiar way of communicating is available, not about factual things, but about feelings.

Presence

There will be times when you believe there is nothing you can do or say to relieve your loved one's psychological or physical pain. When that happens, think about just being present. You'll find many different explanations of what "being present" means. I learned what it meant when I served Emma, whose pain from her lung cancer was only partially controlled. She had abandoned her children for another partner twenty years before and, at the end of her life, regretted the decision. If her increasing pain was to be controlled, her narcotic dosage would have to be substantially increased. Although it would reduce the pain significantly, she decided against it, wanting to be fully conscious as long as possible until she died. Her partner had died a few years back, and her grown children wouldn't talk to her. As much as I wanted to serve her, I didn't know how.

"Emma," I said, "I wish there was something I could do to reduce your pain."

"There is."

"Anything," I said, hoping her answer wouldn't be similar to my first hospice patient's request to end his life.

"Just stay here with me now, and try to be at my side when I die."

As I sat next to her and held her hand, I watched her relax slightly. During each visit for the next three weeks, we would talk until the pain was unbearable. Then, I'd stop speaking and just hold her hand. I wasn't able to be with her when she died, since it occurred suddenly during her sleep. But I think knowing I was willing to be with her at the moment of her death was comforting to her. For me, being present is the willingness to sit silently when there is nothing I can do other than witness someone's pain.

Use Touch to Convey Connectiveness

There is something magical about touch. It forms a physical connection that is important for those who have a progressive illness. There are many things that can make loved ones feel isolated. Few are as pervasive as a debilitating illness. They may look at themselves not only as "different" but also as continually evolving, getting farther and farther away from who they were. And it's not only a self-perception. They experience it when medical personnel focus on the illness as if the label were them, and when friends stop visiting because they don't know how to verbally interact anymore.

When I started hospice volunteer work, I didn't understand the importance of touch, and I remembered the instructions I had given to my student clinicians in the university communicative disorders clinic: "Don't touch the clients, not even children!" It was a particularly litigious period in the 1980s, and accusations of inappropriate touching were rampant. But during my hospice training, we all attended a session where we were taught to use a limited form of massage with our patients. I felt uncomfortable for three reasons. First, I wasn't sure how appropriate it would be, given the decades-old admonitions to my students. Second, touch was something I had avoided in general. And third, I wasn't sure how I would use massage with patients who were dying.

During the training session, the massage therapist explained that we shouldn't think about massage as the type you receive at a spa. Rather, massage for hospice patients was a way of connecting to the person we were serving. She suggested that when we did massage, we try to remember how we would stroke our pets. There is a way we convey love to our animals that is neither learned nor contrived. It's as if we don't need to worry what anyone thinks of us as we display affection — we have no hidden agendas or images we're trying to protect. When we stroke our pets, the only thing we're doing is showing them love. The same honesty can be there when you stroke someone with a progressive illness, whether you're a physician or a friend.

I've always lived with dogs, and even though I understood immediately what the therapist was saying, emotional honesty with an animal is different than with a human being. There is no threat in being open with animals. If they don't accept what you're offering, they don't make you feel bad, or hold it against you, or tell all their friends what a fool you made of yourself. I quickly learned that the same was true of my hospice patients. When I started using therapeutic massage with patients, I began to understand that massage for the dying was about establishing a connection with another human being. I found my hands were capable of expressing feelings I never thought possible: the commonality I felt with a dying person, an understanding of what he or she was experiencing, and my willingness to be present during fear and pain. None of which could be expressed with words.

Music

In his book *This Is Your Brain on Music*, Daniel Levitin presents a compelling argument that, neurologically, our brains are wired to connect more with music than with words. In caregiving, music can be used in four different ways: as a form of entertainment, as a way to tap into memories, as a form of communication that can be used when words can't, and as a way to ease the end of someone's life. The style and form of each is different.

I rarely "entertain" my patients with my music. Frankly, I'm not that good of a musician. I know that inevitably I'll play a wrong note in a song I memorized, or my lack of breath control will result in notes lost. It's not something I think a struggling person wants to hear. Most of what I play for my patients is improvisations on my *shakuhachi* or Native American flute. Since what I play is rarely anything a patient might identity as a familiar tune, my music doesn't offer someone with memory problems an entryway to his past, unless something in my music connects with a similar tune in his memory. What I hope is that my music sets the stage for communicating with a patient when he may no longer understand words, or when a patient is struggling to leave.

I was asked to perform a vigil for a patient I had never met. He lived with his partner of fifteen years in a San Francisco penthouse. After we removed all the items related to his illness, the room was arranged so that treasured items were within his line of sight. When I began playing my Native American flute, the hospice nurse entered the apartment and sat quietly until I finished playing. When I was done, she went to the patient's side.

"Did you like that?" she said. He nodded his head. "Did it take you to someplace special?" Again he nodded. "Where to?" she persisted.

He opened his eyes and said, "I can't tell you, you're not allowed there."

That was the first time I understood the power of music and the place it can have in dying. Since that time, I've reverently played my flutes for patients I believed would benefit from hearing them. Over the years, I've come to learn that some characteristics of music work better than others. Softness in volume is always preferable. Whenever I've offered choices in the range of notes (Native American flutes are each individually tuned), patients have always chosen the lower registers. Slow-moving tunes (either improvised or recognizable ones) are preferable to those with a quicker tempo. Notes that blend into each other have a more calming effect than crisper ones (staccato). Regardless of how much a patient appreciates the music, it seems that twenty minutes is the maximum length of time a patient will want to listen.

If in the course of hospice care I'm able to begin playing my music for patients when they are still cognizant of my presence, I always tell them that there may come a time when my words won't make any sense to them. If that happens, they should just listen to the music and know I'm at their side.

FINAL THOUGHTS

Above all else, communication is the way we manage the world and make sense of it. We use it to request things we would like other people to do, or to tell them things we would like them to understand about what we see and feel. Communication is also talking to ourselves as we explore how we feel about things, what we have done, are doing, or will be doing. We use it to make permanent — via written words — the experiences we want to preserve. Communication is a central feature of our lives, yet we treat it as if it were something very simple.

Over the millennia, humans invented complexities and nuances to enhance communication, from imbedded grammatical structures to sarcasm. And because it is such a marvelous tool, we need not think consciously about it. Trillions of brain cells allow everything to run pretty smoothly, until something goes wrong. Slowly, things begin to crumble. At first there may be minor problems, such as not remembering a name; then, with increasing ferocity, the fundamental blocks of communication begin to fall apart. Words become locked in our minds, refusing to come forth no matter how many tricks we use to coax them out. And if they do reluctantly emerge, they may no longer make sense. When finally we no longer know how to access words, the structure we have based our lives on — one that involves seeing things in words — falls apart, and we are left isolated, not able to tell our caregivers what's wrong or to share with them what we feel. And then, what we do is use any means to say, "Hey,

I'm still here, and I'm afraid." But often our best attempts, those we may struggle with, are misinterpreted as rude or even cruel.

Other forms of communication, such as music and touch, help soothe our feelings and give us some connection with others, but ultimately we remain isolated, waiting for it and us to end.

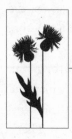

CHAPTER 5

When the Mind Wanders
Aging, Illness, and Dementia

When I said to a friend that I thought some of his father's behaviors indicated dementia, he said, "No, it's not dementia, it's Alzheimer's." He proceeded to go into a long list of diagnostic features distinguishing Alzheimer's from other forms of dementia and memory problems associated with aging and chronic sleep deprivation. I listened patiently during the twenty-minute lecture. Although the lesson was informative, I wondered how knowing the finer distinctions of dementia would change anything in the treatment of his father's problems. There is much interest in developing differential diagnostic tests for various cognitive problems, but much less interest in developing specific strategies for treating their resulting problems.

Knowing the specific medical diagnosis of a memory problem doesn't mean we are limited to a unique strategy for dealing with it. For example, for caregivers it's more important to know how to prevent and deal with disorientation in the middle of a shopping mall, regardless of whether it comes from aging, Alzheimer's, another form of dementia, or chronic sleep deprivation. A number of years ago I went into a huge mall in Phoenix with my son when we were visiting potential colleges for him in Arizona. He went off to look at video games while I entered an office supply store. We were to meet at a specific time at the entrance we had come in. I was having severe sleep problems at that time and had neglected to identify any of the landmarks by the store's entrance. At the appointed time I stood in front of the entrance and waited for my son.

After ten minutes I knew that either something was wrong with him or I wasn't at the right entrance. I looked at the store's map and realized there were ten entrances. I was disoriented, but I also realized that when my son couldn't find me, he would worry. That's when I panicked. What I experienced was similar to what anyone with a memory problem would go through when lost in what should have been a familiar place. It's difficult to describe the feeling of utter helplessness. Fortunately for me, I knew that my difficulties wouldn't lead to more disabling conditions, as happens with dementia. My son found me after I realized that the only thing I could do was stay put. He systematically went to each of the entrances until he found me standing there like a lost child. I realized from the experience that one strategy that would have worked for me would also have worked for anyone with a memory problem — I needed an external mapping system, on a card, which would have allowed me to know where I was and where I should be.

With a general understanding of how normal memory works, we can develop strategies to reduce the problem, whatever the cause. Grouping illnesses like Alzheimer's and Lewy body syndrome with milder forms of memory problems — such as memory dysfunction related to chronic sleep deprivation, and age-related senility — isn't an attempt to equate them. But strategies effective for one can be effective for the others along the severity continuum, with varying degrees of success — strategies effective for Alzheimer's patients can help someone suffering from severe sleep deprivation. The main difference is that, where I might need to use them occasionally, Alzheimer's patients may need them constantly. As one person with Alzheimer's said to me: "I used to have more good days than bad days. Now it's just the opposite."

WHAT'S INVOLVED IN MEMORY?

When we think of memory, we think of something simple, such as bits of information that enter the mind, get stored, and then are, at the appropriate time, regurgitated. But specific things go on inside the brain that cause it to take the information and do incredible things with it. There is still much we don't know about memory, and much of what we do know is the result of indirect evidence: we have created theories based on how well our memory works or falls apart. At its most basic level, memory requires four steps: attention, understanding, storage, and retrieval. And putting them all together is called "executive functioning," a fancy phrase meaning that the brain manipulates all four aspects to do something, say, cook an omelet. This is similar to the way an executive directs his staff. Four separate steps, and something to organize them. A hiccup in any step or in how your loved one coordinates them can lead to memory problems. Neurologists and neuropsychologists may find this explanation simplistic. But it's functional, allowing anyone who daily cares for someone else with memory impairments to understand what to do when, for example, a loved one forgets how to put on a shirt or thinks that a strange person is in the house.

Executive Functioning

Executive functioning is a technical phrase that describes how the brain moves information around to get something done. Think of cooking. You have a recipe, you know the number of servings you want to make, and you've purchased all the items you'll need. Although all these things appears to be connected, they aren't, really, until you start measuring, preparing, and cooking the items. Executive functioning is what you do to make the meal.

Anyone with experience in a kitchen knows that to make a meal you must do specific things. You look at the recipe and it says, "Beat two eggs until frothy." You put down the recipe book, get two eggs from the refrigerator, find a suitable bowl, and crack the eggs into it. Then you find a whisk and beat them. But where did the knowledge of how to beat eggs come from? It came from long-term memory — the repository of things you learned a while ago and keep in storage until you need them. Executive functioning grabs that knowledge from long-term memory, along with the recipe's components held in short-term memory, and does its magic. And, behold, you've made the perfect omelet.

A loved one who has problems with executive functioning may appear confused while doing even the simplest things. The problem may not have anything to do with remembering something; it may have to do with how to use those memories. A friend of mine who has Alzheimer's told me about an incident where he was at the edge of a curb and, for an instant, didn't remember how to ascend it. Fortunately for him, this episode ended quickly. An example of a problem related to short-term memory, rather than executive functioning, is what happens to me when my sleep deprivation becomes acute and I try to move a paragraph from one place in a document to another. I cut a paragraph, but before pasting it I forget what I copied, even though only seconds have passed.

One strategy to use with executive functioning disorders is to graphically reproduce the steps involved in an action. One caregiver placed numbered and color-coded symbols on kitchen cabinets for her mother. In cabinet 1 were plates. In cabinet 2 was the cereal. On the outside of the refrigerator, and on the carton of milk, the daughter wrote the number 3. On the kitchen table she put a picture of someone pouring cereal into a bowl, pouring in milk, and then eating it. She knew that by following the numbers, her mother could prepare her own breakfast.

Attention

Attention is more complicated than most of us realize. We may assume loved ones just need to listen or watch, but what does listening and watching require? Loved ones must extract what's important from everything else. That's as true for someone with dementia as it is for a COPD patient struggling for every breath. In an earlier chapter, I noted the role that noise, pain, and emotions play in how loved ones function. Anything that interferes with concentration can affect attention. Say a caregiver is leaving instructions telling her loved one which pills to take while she is out. She believes her instructions are so simple that he will have no problem with them. But while she is outlining them, her loved one's intense pain surfaces, blotting out everything, including those simple instructions.

You can try several different strategies to increase your loved one's attention. I presented some of these in chapter 4, such as minimizing noise. If you want her to pay attention, turn off all media. Another strategy is to highlight what you want her to notice by saying something like: "This is important." You can also increase your volume level to emphasize this importance. And you can pare down the information to just the important aspects of your message.

Deciding what works is more art and observation than science. I've found persistence to be a more valuable asset than perfection. There will be few instances when you can do everything perfectly. But you can always persist, getting better and closer to your ultimate goal. When I work on memory with chronically or terminally ill patients, I assume I'll likely get it wrong the first time — and maybe even the second or third time. I don't get upset, nor do I see it as failure. I developed some of my most useful techniques after getting things wrong numerous times with patients. It's like starting at the base of a pyramid. At the bottom are many possibilities, but as you ascend, the options become fewer, until you reach the pinnacle.

Don't feel bad if you, too, make mistakes. Professionals make as many as you do, even if they're reluctant to admit it.

Understanding

When a person with a progressive illness pays attention to something, he may initially understand it. But as the information piles up, he may seem to understand less and less. This may be caused by one of two different problems. First, the information may be using up his capacity for executive functioning. The person listens to what is being said and understands it, but as the conversation goes on, his executive functioning eventually fatigues, making it difficult to move the information into short-term memory. It stays in working memory, simply occupying space and never moving on, or maybe it just drops out. It's almost as if you have been listening to a lecture for forty-five minutes. When the presenter began, you were able to understand everything. But since he's incredibly boring, you find that, as he continues talking, it takes an ever-increasing effort to understand what he is saying. The same thing may happen to your loved one, but instead of forty-five minutes, it may take only ten. And instead of a boring lecturer, the speaker could be a friend or a professional talking about something of little interest to your loved one. Second, executive functioning may, for some reason, get stuck processing one thing and be unable to move on to the next. Imagine that you are playing the best tennis game of your life. You look at your watch and see that in thirty minutes you have an appointment across town. If you immediately stop, you can still make it. But the intoxication of the game is so great that you decide to delay. You'll just be late. A similar process may be occurring in your loved one. You've just finished discussing an important financial issue with him and are explaining the schedule for the day. You assume he has been listening, since he nodded his head at every point. When you move toward the door to leave — something you just discussed with him

— he looks at you blankly and says, "Where are you going?" He isn't consciously ignoring the schedule; his mind may be stuck on the financial issue.

We don't know which, if either, of the two explanations is correct, but intuitively, it seems that something like this is occurring. In any case, caregivers can focus on figuring out what may contribute to a loved one's difficulty. Decide what can most easily be controlled. In this case, it's the amount of incoming information. When we talk to our loved ones, we often provide more information than they need. In normal conversations, the extra information serves as connective tissue holding together ideas and conveying warmth and affection — all important things for a relationship. But when extra information is interspersed between specific instructions, a person with a memory problem may miss the central message. When my wife is explaining something to me, and I get the central theme, I'll often say, "I've got it," and reiterate what she has asked me to do. That's our sign for her to stop giving me information. I know that, with my sleep deprivation, the more information I receive, the less I'll retain.

Storage and Retrieval

Storage is something we can know about only indirectly. We assume our loved ones store new information, but we have no direct knowledge of it until they attempt to retrieve it. Problems in retrieval may relate mainly to how the information was saved. The mind does strange things with the information it receives. We think that memory is stored chemically, and that different parts of what one attempts to remember are stored in different parts of the brain. For example, your loved one is in the doctor's office and is receiving updated information on her condition. The doctor is explaining how her ALS is progressing and points to a chart showing the degeneration of the synaptic connections; each depiction is labeled.

The entire explanation lasts five minutes. The mind takes the whole interaction and stores the doctor's words in one area of the brain, the written words somewhere else, and the graphic representations in a third area. And let's throw in a peculiar smell that permeates the office. That's stored somewhere else. Evidence suggests that there may even be redundancy (the same information is stored in multiple locations). The next week, you ask your loved one how much she remembers of the visit. To retrieve it, her brain now has to put everything back together. She may be unable to access all the elements, but if she can access enough of them, she will remember the interaction, if not completely, then partially.

But what happens if the initial setting for receiving the information isn't as rich as the one I just described? Let's say the information is conveyed via telephone, where only the words are available to constitute the entire memory. If the area responsible for storing words is damaged, little is left for the brain to use for retrieving the memory. That's why making the initial setting rich, but not overly complicated, will enhance your loved one's memory, regardless of the degree of impairment. For example, instead of just telling your loved one what she should do when you are out, demonstrate each step of it. Initially, loved ones may act negatively. One person said, "I'm not that stupid yet, I can understand the words." But understanding is not the issue. Providing the brain with multiple ways of storing information about a specific event may make it easier to retrieve the instruction's steps. When I don't have access to my iPhone or pen and paper, and I'm trying to store information, I often mentally form a picture of it, repeatedly constructing it until I feel I've moved it into short-term memory, where hopefully it will stay until I can jot it down.

Pumping Up Plasticity

Plasticity, according to neuroscientists, is the ability of the brain to build new synaptic connections between neurons in response to learning. We knew this was important in how children learn, but believed that it didn't occur in adults with Alzheimer's or other dementias. In Alzheimer's and other dementias, the connections break, which results in memory problems. But new research shows that in dementia patients, new synaptic connections can be grown.

Does this mean that learning new things can stop or reverse dementia? Maybe not stop, but definitely slow down. My friend Norm McNamara, author of *Me and My Alzheimer's*, was unable to use his computer for three weeks. During this period, his wife noticed a reduction in his speech ability and general orientation. When he again went online, his granddaughter, who was watching him type, pointed out that what he had just written made no sense. He realized that even a small amount of inactivity substantially reduced his functioning. After again using his computer to write articles, correspond with friends, and gather information, he found his abilities had returned.

The lesson for caregivers is that we can use the brain's ability to create new synaptic connections to slow down the inevitable results of dementia, probably not via rote memory exercises but by learning something new. In the past, when I practiced playing my Native American flute and *shakuhachi*, I focused on endlessly playing the same tunes until I got them as close to perfect as I could. My playing of those tunes improved, but my overall musical skill didn't. However, when I started improvising — trying to put together unique musical phrases — I noticed that my overall playing improved. Help your loved one engage in new activities within her comfort level.

Commercially available programs may help with this, but life is filled with so many possibilities that you can probably construct your own activities from what you already have in your home. And there are advantages in doing so. First of all, you can relate an exercise directly to issues that are problematic for your loved one. Devise an activity, for example, to help her remember where things are placed in the house. Take several items from around your home and place them on the kitchen table. Then ask your loved one to help you put them away. The activity of putting them where they belong isn't as important as your loved one's explanation of why they go there. That, I believe, is fertile ground for growing new synaptic connections.

A second reason for real-life activities is that they are less likely to become boring. For example, when you walk in a new area, ask your loved one to talk about what he or she is seeing as you stroll along. It never gets boring if you continually find new areas to walk.

A third reason is that real-life activities create more of the memory hooks that are used for retrieval. Looking at a program on a computer screen will create far fewer of these hooks than gardening in the backyard, with its abundant colors, smells, and textures. Finally, and perhaps most important, real-life activities become generalizable, which means what was learned in one activity can be used in other, similar ones. For example, the skills your loved one uses to orient herself in a supermarket can also be used in a department store. The possibilities for creating real-life activities are endless. And when it comes to memory problems, sitting and doing nothing may speed up the loss of function.

Anchoring Memory

Arguing with someone who can't retrieve a memory is like telling a blind person he should be able to distinguish between red and green. When someone insists that I should be able to remember an event that has permanently entered a sinkhole in my memory, I eventually agree and say, "Of course, I remember it now," having no recollection of it. I know the event is permanently gone, but it's difficult to convince someone without a memory problem that, even with clues, it can't be retrieved. Don't insist he should be able to remember, and don't become angry when he can't.

As your loved one's ability to remember fades, provide strategies for enhancing the probability that a current event will be remembered.

For example, when I was visiting one of my hospice patients with dementia, she would be annoyed with me, saying, "You didn't come last week like you promised." I never missed a session with her. The solution was to have her circle the day of my next visit and have her caretaker cross off days as my visit approached. Although she couldn't remember circling the date, she knew she had done it. The loss of memory is incredibly depressing. It not only deprives a loved one of the past but also signals that one of the most important parts of being human is dissolving. Allowing loved ones to hold on to that ability as long as possible gives them the feeling of still being connected.

STABILITY

When we think about helping our loved ones to remember, we may think especially about the internal aspects of what is required to communicate. But there are also other, external aspects that you can adjust.

Keep the House Organized

I was concerned one day when I came home and couldn't find my mother. The back of the house has a steep bank below the deck that leads to a forested area. When I saw that the gate to the stairs was open, my concern turned to panic. At that time she was in her mid-sixties and often became confused when situations or discussions were anything other than linear. I raced down the stairs expecting the worst. There, I saw her emerging from a stand of trees, carrying a handful of leaves and twigs, smiling as if she had just solved a complex puzzle.

"Mom, what are you doing?" I asked.

"Straightening out the forest."

When she saw my bewildered look, she explained. "From inside the house, it looked so messy. I thought it would be nice to clean it up a little."

"But, Mom," I said, "it's a forest." She stared at me as if I just couldn't understand what she was saying. And she was right.

Now, more than twenty years after she died, I think I finally understand. I believe I confused "just being Mom" with the early signs of dementia. She died from a heart attack before her symptoms could develop into anything definitive. As I deal with an increasing number of hospice patients with Alzheimer's and other forms of dementia, I think back to my mother's efforts at tidying up the forest. I've come to realize that the need for structure increases as those elements that we have been using to make sense of our lives disappear.

I've seen families and health care staff misinterpret older people's behaviors, or the behaviors of people who are near death, as the inexplicable result of "losing their minds." These family members and staff did not understand that what they saw might have been an attempt to regain the structure that had allowed them to map out what was familiar in their lives. With various forms of dementia and many terminal illnesses, the ground — the base that allows people to know where and who they are — continually shifts, though it pauses occasionally and gives them a false sense that the frightening progression has finally stopped. Straightening out the forest is just another way of making the ground shake less.

The Endless Repetition of Questions

I've found that when loved ones with various forms of dementia begin repeating the same question or asking multiple questions that are very similar — especially after having received an answer — their specific concerns may indicate something general about the illness's progression. Repeatedly asking if he is going to the senior center that day may be a person's expression of the fear that the structural templates in his mind aren't working. What I've seen in most patients is that the greater the loss of the internal structure, the more frightening the world becomes and the more repetitive questions become.

I often see caregivers misinterpret the intent of questions. To understand what is happening, write down each question your loved one asks and look for commonalities in them. For example, questions about where someone else is don't necessarily mean your loved one is concerned about that person. They may instead indicate he is beginning to lose the connection between people and places. If that is your conclusion, devise a strategy to connect people and places — for example, show him a picture of his aunt outside her house in Detroit. Attaching pictures of family members and their locations to a piece of poster board may be helpful. Glue pieces of Velcro to the pictures of individual family members and to the poster board, and then you can move these people around between locations. This works especially well if many people are located in the same city and it's just the location within the city that keeps changing. For example, if you're leaving for an hour to go to the store while someone watches your husband, place your picture on the store. If you and other family members travel between two or more cities, you can divide the poster into sections.

What to Do When Few Words Are Left

There may come a time when your loved one can no longer use words. That doesn't mean she doesn't understand all communication. It means it's time to initiate a simplified communication device — perhaps pictures that express feelings and needs. There are many available for purchase, so you won't need to construct your own. More sophisticated hardware and software are available for computers. Regardless of the type of alternative communication you choose, it's important to introduce it before you need it.

You may find it helpful to contact faculty members at a local university who specialize in alternative or augmentative communication before you speak with representatives of companies that make specific devices. The differences between devices can be complicated, and you're more likely to receive an unbiased review of them from someone who has no financial interest in your decision. Some loved ones may be initially averse to using one, especially when verbal communication is still possible. Accepting the device means accepting a dreadful part of the disease. And this may require an extensive amount of compassionate discussion.

That was the case with an ALS patient who, since he could still mouth words, refused to communicate his needs by writing them on paper. When he lost the ability to form words and had limited fine motor control over his hands and fingers, he insisted on using a regular pen instead of an assistive grip pen that would have given him more control. When he had only limited gross control over his arms, he wouldn't try an electronic communicator. With any progressive disease, you should always focus on what your loved one will be able to do next month, rather than today. As depressing as it may be for him to look into the future, learning new skills ahead of time, while he still has the capability, will lessen the anxiety he will feel later when few choices are left.

We often look for ways to enable our loved ones to communicate just as they did before becoming ill. As a caregiver, you should change your mind-set and think in the simplest terms — what does my loved one need to communicate the basics about her needs and feelings? One ALS patient insisted on using complete sentences rather than just the basics to communicate with me when using her eye-gazing software. Eye-gazing software allows people to select letters, words, and phrases just by gazing at them on a computer screen. The more complete her sentences were, the more time it took my patient to communicate her thoughts, and the fewer ideas we exchanged. Even when I orally completed her sentences as the first few words appeared on the computer screen, she wouldn't stop. I would have to wait until every word was spelled out. And if she made a typing error, she would move the cursor back to the misspelled word and rewrite it with the correct spelling. Eventually I realized it was more important for her to retain this pre-ALS skill than to discuss a greater number of ideas. Yet for another ALS patient, telegraphic speech (leaving out everything that wasn't necessary for understanding the meaning) allowed him to discuss a multitude of needs with his caregiver.

Confusing Emotions, Physiology, and Overloads

As a loved one's illness progresses, the term *cognitive problem* is often tossed around, as if those strange things said and done are just part of a loved one's "losing his mind." The cause may indeed be the physiological deterioration of the brain, but it can also be pain, overmedication, or too much stimuli. The uncertainty of coming to terms with one's life near its end can be misidentified as an indication of dementia. Also, the added time required to process information as one ages can be misidentified as a sign of a cognitive disorder, which it may not be. For example, I find that it sometimes takes me a bit longer to transfer an idea onto paper — but I would take umbrage if someone thought my slowness was the first sign of dementia.

The problem of misdiagnosing behaviors is not merely speculative. For example, I have seen many individuals in hospice care whose slowness in responding, or whose disconnected discourse, was treated as if it signaled Alzheimer's or another form of dementia. It didn't, but was instead an expression of their difficulty in formulating thoughts when pain became all-consuming.

Exceeding Thresholds

A loved one is taxed both physically and emotionally with the onset of any illness. What someone was able to do prior to the onset, she may not be able to do afterward. My wife experienced this after her stroke. Her problem was that her threshold, the point beyond which the body or mind doesn't work effectively, was lowered. With my wife, one trigger that lowered her threshold was insufficient sleep. Some of my patients' thresholds were triggered by too much information, which reduced their ability to make decisions. Some could no longer deal with the world when a certain level of anxiety or stress was exceeded. But in every case, when their stress or anxiety dropped back below the threshold, their behaviors and thinking either became normal or were vastly improved.

In thinking about your loved one's threshold, try to identify the times when you think he exceeds it. As he approaches his threshold, you'll see changes — it usually is not a matter of being fine one minute and incapacitated the next. Look for what occurs simultaneously with the changes. Are too many activities taking place? Has the noise level increased substantially? Is your loved one being asked to do something he feels he can't? Whatever it is, it may be his trigger, something to avoid in the future. And it may not be any one thing, but rather a series of them — for example, a visit by an insensitive relative after a poor night's sleep on a day when the dosage of his medicine is increased. Often, a threshold may be exceeded and a behavior triggered before you can prevent it from happening. But the sooner you can change the circumstances that triggered him, the quicker the recovery. For some patients, rest or sleep does wonders. For others, the elimination of stressful activities does it. You'll need to experiment. Understand that once a threshold has been exceeded, you may need to make choices for your loved one. During the first three months of my wife's recovery, I would have to insist that she stop trying to put things away and rest. She didn't realize she wasn't functioning well. With time, she was able to monitor herself.

Some Practical Ways to Monitor Wandering

A loved one's wandering within or outside of the home can be a concern for caregivers. Some facilities use sophisticated entry and exit devices, which can consist of coded locks, alarms, and computer alerts, to mention just a few features. Some of these devices may not be appropriate or may be too expensive for caregivers to install in the home. However, some useful and inexpensive devices are available. For example, you might want to invest in an inexpensive home monitoring system that will allow you, while you're away from home, to watch specific rooms or doors via the Web. There are smartphone applications that make this possible by sending you motion-detection and audio alerts while you're away. You also can equip your home with an inexpensive closed-circuit monitoring system, with cameras located at the most critical parts of your house, and alarm the exterior doors.

FINAL THOUGHTS

The scientist in me tells me to look for the orderly and precise way memories are lost in my patients. After all, if I can just identify *exactly* what isn't happening, maybe I can develop strategies that will always accommodate their illnesses. Unfortunately, my simplistic hope is rarely fulfilled. When researchers try to map out the problems of a system that they only theoretically understand, what they develop is a set of guesses that sometimes work, but which at other times fail miserably.

When I asked Rick Phelps, the founder of Memory People, who has early-onset Alzheimer's disease, if any of the published programs designed to improve memory in people with Alzheimer's disease were effective, he said none that he had tried helped. While they all contained wonderful steps to improve memory, or they attempted to delay the ravages of Alzheimer's, none could help him find his car in the Wal-Mart parking lot. The reality of what he faces every day contains more variables than the most sophisticated program can handle. For Rick, as parts of his memory dropped out — whether they involved short-term memory, long-term memory, or executive functioning — the holes became too immense to fill, regardless of what was suggested by well-meaning friends and professionals. And what was left for both him and his wife was acceptance.

Dallas Shieck, another person with early-onset Alzheimer's and a gifted writer, expressed in an Alzheimer's support-group chat room on the Internet what she felt when the holes became deeper and wider.

> *Life seems to speed to a conclusion I am unaware of, yet I re-mind myself there is actually very little in life we can ever truly be sure of. It is crazy to try. Maybe Alzheimer's is a way for God to remind us He is the one in control. Thoughts enter my head and drift so freely they are difficult to catch. I have no net any-more that will keep them from escaping. It has grown quite tat-tered from so much use lately. I never needed it so much as I have these last few years.*
>
> *I am haunted by something I do not comprehend, struggle to find something I cannot remember having lost or even what it might have been. Also I realize I am losing myself, little by little, and am quite beyond recall. Night dreams blend into day-dreams and into what reality there might be. What thoughts I have are often in pieces before they reach the page, whether I attempt to type or write with a pen. Where will I be when all is said and done? My life was such that all I ever had were dreams, never a true opportunity to reach for them, to fulfill them.*
>
> *Now I stand unsteadily on the edge of a void of which very soon there will be no return. I weep, but not for me, I weep for those I leave behind because I leave them and am still here for them to see, but not to interact with. I weep, not for me, there is no point. I weep for thought that has tried so hard to reach the page, to be shared, to reach out to others, but has become lost or scattered, or shattered.*
>
> *I have been admired for my strength, yet have always felt*

so very weak and foolish, so very unworthy of admiration, of af-
fection, of notice of any kind. I am a mere mortal slowly being
emptied of life, of thought, of being. Anything I brought with me
into this world I will take with me. But I will try to leave behind
a greater love than I take and hope there is peace for all. Now
my thoughts are becoming muddled, so I must say good night.

As caregivers, all we can do is bear witness to what our loved
ones are experiencing, knowing that sometimes the only thing we
can offer is our compassion. In this chapter, I've made no distinctions between types of memory problems by diagnostic categories.
I've done so for a number of reasons. The first is that memory problems tend to be progressive. So what isn't a problem today may
become one tomorrow. And categorically stating, "This is Alzheimer's," may not be accurate, especially if it's early in its onset or the
problems tend to come and go. Also, understanding the components
of memory will enable you, as a caregiver, to have a more pragmatic
view of the problems and, more important, to begin designing strategies that, though they do not correct the problems, can at least make
your loved one's life easier.

Neurologists and neuropsychologists will probably think this
chapter offers a simplistic explanation of how the mind works. However, caregivers need, not theories, but practical things they can do
when their loved ones experience a specific problem. Finding strategies for memory problems is often a trial-and-error process, especially when the symptoms aren't always present. It's always best to
err on the side of caution, in the same way that you would install a
burglar alarm "just in case." If you are using strategies that may not
be necessary, the worst that can happen is nothing. I may remember a
meeting without looking at my iPhone calendar, but it's nice to know
the information will be available if the "fog" rolls in. Putting strategies in place will give your loved one the greatest opportunity for
reducing the anxiety and pain a memory disorder inevitably creates.

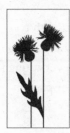

CHAPTER 6

When a Loved One's Death Is Close, and Afterward

There is a twilight quality that develops as a loved one's death nears. The air reminds me of the crispness I've experienced at the beginning of a thunderstorm. The experience is different when it occurs in the quietness of one's home, surrounded by family and friends, not in a sterile hospital room with a never-ending stream of medical staff and the constant beeping of monitoring devices. Dying is tumultuous. You may not see anything chaotic externally, but internally the body and mind are engaged in an extreme marathon. Physically, systems are no longer acting as they used to. Emotionally, the person is contending with a past possibly filled with regrets and unfinished business, and a future that she knows will not happen. And you may be responsible for "managing" this profound event.

Most of the comments in this chapter apply to dying at home or in a compassionate care facility, but not in a hospital. It's been my experience with both patients and my own relatives that, until recently, hospitals have not offered the type of death I believe most people want to experience. Some progressive hospitals understand this and have set aside areas where patients, attended by their family and friends, can experience a more peaceful death.

THE LOOSE ENDS

As death becomes imminent, loved ones may be consumed with trying to tie up the loose ends of their lives. Some things are easy to complete, such as thanking caregivers and friends for everything they have done. Other things, like asking for forgiveness for past unskillful acts, are more difficult.

A Good-Bye Party

One of the first things Gene did when I entered his apartment was to show me the chair Tennessee Williams sat in when they discussed the state of theater in San Francisco.

"We were good friends," he said. "Well, maybe not friends, but colleagues. I'm sure if he were still alive he would be at my good-bye party." Gene was a well-known actor in San Francisco and was dying of liver cancer.

He told me about a huge affair being organized by friends, colleagues, and the many fellow actors he had helped throughout the years. "Why should my friends celebrate my life when I'm not there?" he asked. The planning started when he received a terminal prognosis. Because Gene had been an actor for sixty years, the event had to be choreographed as meticulously as if it were opening night on Broadway. And, of course, he expected me to be there. One week later I entered the lobby of a theater in which he had often performed. After elaborate trays of food and many glasses of champagne had been served, his closest friends went to his side and told him how much he meant to them, and how he had contributed to their lives. Most were local actors, but a few I recognized from films and television. There was weeping throughout the conversations, but these were expressions of gratitude for having been allowed into the life of this wonderful person. During the time I served him afterward, he often retold the events that occurred at the party, marveling at how fulfilling his life had been.

A good-bye party is a glorious event celebrating life, and it gives permission for people important in your loved one's life to say good-bye, an act that is difficult for many to do. The good-bye party says to those who attend: "I know I'm dying, and I want an opportunity to tell you how much you've meant to me. And you have my permission to do the same." People who have attended such parties rank them with some of the most meaningful and joyous events in their lives.

Grant a Last Wish

Life can be celebrated in many ways. One patient talked about her "bucket list," which involved first-class travel to places she'd always wanted to visit with her husband, who had died a few years before her diagnosis. Other patients decided to take time to appreciate the environment that surrounded them. One patient, whose beautiful backyard had been ignored for years because he was too busy to experience it, started each day by sipping coffee alone among the rose bushes. Whether these celebrations are as simple as quietly contemplating one's life in the backyard or as expensive as booking the best cabin on a cruise ship, they are all appropriate. Bill's approach was one that I could relate to. After his laryngectomy (removal of the voice box), doctors found that the cancer had spread to his chest. According to him, his brain was next. At our first meeting, I talked and he wrote:

"I don't think I have much time left."

"Why do you think that?" I said.

"I can feel something different is going on inside me."

He was aware of the mucous coming out of his stoma (a hole in the front of his throat through which he breathed) and constantly dabbed at it, gesturing an apology to me each time he did it.

"It's all right," I said. "I was a speech-language pathologist before retiring, and I treated people who had laryngectomies."

"I still feel bad about it," he wrote. "I'm embarrassed."

That was how our conversation began during the first ten minutes of my visit. Bill had few friends, and his remaining family members were somewhere back East. He had had no contact with them for many years, and when asked if he wanted us to find them, he said no. He had no idea where they lived and even if he'd known, they wouldn't remember him. I'm not sure what triggered the next conversation; maybe it was my saying that I too had had cancer, or maybe because instead of asking questions, I allowed him to lead the conversation. He said he knew his life was coming to an end. Looking around his room, I saw nothing of a personal nature other than a picture of him smiling and wearing a San Francisco Giants baseball jacket and cap. He told me it was taken when he was celebrating a Giants win over the Dodgers. He pointed to the picture and then himself, and shook his head. The person in the picture was robust, happy, and fit looking. In person, Bill could have been mistaken for a concentration camp survivor.

I was at a loss to provide him with anything to make his death easier. I don't know why I said it, but I asked if there was anything he wanted to do before he died. He thought for a few minutes and then wrote, "Go fishing." I said that it might take a while to arrange it, but I would see what I could do. I would be visiting him in a week, and if possible, we would go on our trip then. It would take some planning, since Bill was weak and needed a wheelchair, an oxygen tank, a portable suction machine, and vials of a morphine derivative he could orally ingest if his breathing became too difficult or his neck pain too severe. As I left, I asked the nurse how much time she thought he had left.

"Yesterday I would have said at least a few months. But he doesn't look very well today. Maybe a few weeks."

I found a wheelchair ramp when I arrived at the lake in San Francisco where Bill told me he had fished for years. From the car I called the hospice: "Tell Bill I'll see him in two days." When I arrived two days later, the nurse told me they weren't able to wake him. I sat with him for a while before putting pictures on the bulletin board next to his bed of me fishing in the marshes of Louisiana and in the Grand Canyon. I also left two articles I had written on saltwater fly-fishing. We would try again the next week. When I arrived the following week, I found Bill propped up in bed. He pointed to the pictures. "I looked at them every day and also read the articles," he wrote. According to the nurse, every day he'd had her cross out a day on his wall calendar. He had written "Fishing with Stan" on one date and circled it.

We didn't catch any fish at the lake, but that was irrelevant. My final gift to him began the day I told him about our trip. At the lake, I took several pictures of him fishing. When I dropped him off at the hospice, I told him I would bring the pictures in the next day. When I arrived he was again unresponsive. Before leaving, I put fifteen pictures on the wall, the bulletin board, and his tray table, so that if he did wake, he would see a record of his last wish. According to the nurse, they were the last things he looked at before smiling and peacefully slipping into his final coma.

A loved one may ask you to help him fulfill a final request. Or, when you know he feels comfortable discussing it, you can ask him if there is anything he would like to do before he dies. If he has already talked to you about his death and is actively discussing it with you, then that will probably be the time to ask him about his final wish. The words you use should be as simple as those I used with Bill: "Is there something you would like to do that we can start planning for before you die?" Some final requests have seemed strange. One hospice patient asked me to make him a very fatty corned beef sandwich. The request had less to do with the flavor than with reliving the years he had spent in Manhattan with his wife, frequenting the best delicatessens on the Lower East Side. Although last requests may be literal expressions of wanting to again experience a specific activity, they often are attempts to re-create wonderful past emotions.

The celebration of life can involve conversations about the past, developing a journal for friends and future generations (dictated to you, or audio- or videotaped), a visit to a favorite place, eating a favorite food, or even throwing a good-bye party. Regardless of the celebration's form, it allows your loved one to bring into the present the things in his past that made life worthwhile.

Letting Go

We seem to spend our lives holding on to emotions and desires that no longer make any sense. If we could isolate them, as if we were placing a toxic material in a sealed jar, that would be fine. We'd live with them, knowing they were always there but sealed off from our everyday lives. That rarely happens. The emotions we are left with after a negative event stay with us and permeate our lives. As your loved one prepares to die, more than one of these "toxic" memories may surface.

Often this kind of memory has something to do with regretting something one did, or being the victim of an injustice. I've found that when it's possible to let go, it often involves forgiving someone for an unkind act, or being forgiven for a reprehensible act. In past chapters, I've discussed the importance of forgiving and being forgiven. It's never more urgent than close to the end of a loved one's life.

Create a Calm Environment

You can control what's happening around your loved one. The less external agitation there is, the easier it will be for her to deal with what's happening internally. Surround your loved one with peaceful and comforting objects, music, and smells, such as pictures of favorite places, awards commemorating achievements, favorite items, meditative music, and flowers. If possible, remove objects related to her illness. Your ability to anticipate problems well before it's necessary may make it easier for you to create a calm environment. A man with terminal prostate cancer had planned on being cared for by his son and daughter-in-law in their home. It was a large and elegant house that they had started to remodel before my patient knew he was dying. His son also had two teenagers and a five-year-old child. Although my patient had his own room, the environment was so hectic that both he and his son decided the chaos would not permit a peaceful exit. He moved to a hospice.

Where to Stay in Time

However my patients related to the past or future, what became apparent as they neared death was that the more they consciously resided in the present, the easier their deaths were. Grace had always felt very comfortable talking to me about the wonderful experiences she'd had with her husband, who had died ten years earlier. They'd had a glorious life with much love; according to Grace, "We lived fully." But as she came closer to dying, her focus shifted to the future and the experiences she wouldn't have with her grandchildren. The family had always been very open about her condition, especially with her grandchildren, who adored her. And despite her pain, she was trying to stay as long as possible for them.

"Mom," her daughter said to her one day, "I know you're ready to go and are only staying for Sarah and Jim. I want you to know that they have become who you wanted them to be. In them, I see you and all the wonderful things you and Dad taught them. They'll be fine. You gave them everything they will ever need."

Grace seemed to relax. What her daughter had done was pull her consciousness away from the future, with all the regrets it engendered, back into the present, where love was abundant. I believe this shift made it easier for Grace to leave. A simple guideline is to make your loved one's death easier by moving her consciousness as much as possible into the present. In the present, she can prepare for her death by relishing what she did, correcting unskillful acts, and relinquishing the future.

Accept Private Experiences

Sometimes, weeks or days before their deaths, loved ones want to talk about visits they have had from someone who is now dead and who had been close to them. Occasionally, the visitor might be a stranger. My patients have seen relatives, good friends, strangers, and even people in authoritative positions, but no white lights, which are often written about. Many insist that the visit didn't occur during sleep, and that if it did, they were awakened by it. Regardless of when it happened, they assured me, it was real.

There is a debate between members of the spiritual community and neuroscientists about the visitations that dying people report. Neuroscientists offer explanations related to what happens to the brain as neurons begin dying and synaptic connections break. They say that the experiences may appear to be real, but that they are just hallucinations caused by chemical reactions. Those in the spiritual community aren't quick to agree. They concur that some delusions, such as the sense of being locked up in a jail, may derive from the brain's reactions to a toxic chemical generated by the illness. But they also feel that similarities between the stories told by dying people make scientific explanations questionable. A reoccurring theme is that of someone who appears to lead them on a journey — not necessarily to a spiritual place — but on some sort of trip. And the experience is rarely frightening.

It makes little difference where you place yourself in this debate. The discussion may be academic for you, but for your loved one the experience is real. And that's the only thing that matters. If he wants to talk about a visitation, he knows he's risking being labeled as delusional. But he's doing it anyway because he trusts you to understand its importance. Regardless of whether you believe it's a true spiritual event or just the result of dying neurons, be accepting of the experience.

Don't Grieve Excessively in Front of Loved Ones

There is a difference between grieving the eventual loss of a person's life and overtly demonstrating grief in that person's presence. Excessive emotional displays can make death less peaceful. One woman was distraught as her husband drew close to death. His heart had been failing for a number of years, and despite numerous events that could have led to his death, he had persisted. "I have to stay here for her," he said to me. Their relationship had been symbiotic. Each was the other's best friend, and they had been together almost twenty-four hours a day, even before he became ill. Losing Phil would mean that Jenny's life would be halved. Just before he began actively dying, Jenny recognized that this time would most likely be different from all the past critical episodes. Her grief was overwhelming, and she repeatedly pleaded, "Don't leave, honey. Don't leave, I'm not ready." As he struggled to continue breathing, Jenny poured out her grief in his presence. Her son gently led her out of the room and tried to explain to her that Phil, who was probably in great pain, might be staying just for her. And that if she loved him, she would give him permission to leave. She did, and later that day Phil died.

It's natural to grieve the eventual loss of a person and tell him how much he has meant and how much he will be missed. But overtly demonstrating your grief in his presence will make his death, which is certain, become drawn out and possibly result in continued pain. Grieve, but don't allow your feelings of loss to upset the person who is dying. He has more than enough to contend with.

Don't Argue

The person who is dying is juggling many things, some of which are family issues. There are few things as disconcerting to a dying person as witnessing an argument between family members. Occasionally, I've suggested that friends and family members continue their discussion outside the patient's room. One patient of mine who was dying received a visit from her two daughters, neither of whom had previously visited the woman during her illness. My patient had told me that their family had always been dysfunctional. During her daughters' formative years, her husband had left them, and she had been responsible for raising the two girls by herself while working. Eventually, she had become very successful, and so her estate was large. The daughters thought they would inherit everything, and as their mother began actively dying, they discussed the disposition of various pieces of furniture. The discussions turned into arguments that were clearly distressing to my patient. When I suggested that the discussion be taken outside, the daughters ignored me. It was only after my patient began to cry that they stopped.

Always make the assumption that your loved one can hear you right up to the moment of her death, and that what she would have been upset to hear when she was in good health is significantly more distressful as she approaches death. Dying doesn't translate into invisibility.

Accept the Decision to Stop Eating and Drinking

It's natural to want to suggest or even insist that a dying person eat or drink "to keep up his strength," despite his insistence that he isn't hungry or thirsty. As the body begins to shut down, it no longer requires nourishment. Food at this point won't prolong a loved one's life. In fact, the ingestion of food or water may be painful. Accept his decision to stop eating and drinking, and keep all food and food smells out of the room. Many of my patients complained that the smell of food, even foods they had relished throughout their lives, made them nauseous as they came closer to death.

The decision to stop eating and drinking doesn't always mean that death will occur soon. It may be a few days or weeks away. But when death occurs, it's not caused by starvation; the illness has run its course. The loss of appetite is an indication that the body is having difficulty processing food and liquid. The discomfort you may see is not caused by a lack of food but by the disease process. Any dryness of the mouth and lips can be remedied by a sponge paddle (a short stick with a piece of sponge on the end that is dipped in water).

Forgiving

The pain from the past that people experience often follows them to their deaths. I had been visiting Vince weekly for five months, and every week he began by telling me about his distaste for his brother, whom he hadn't spoken to in twenty years. His animosity had to do with a birthday party his brother had decided not to attend. It was Vince's fiftieth birthday, and the entire family had decided to have a huge celebration. A hall was secured, a band was hired, and an expensive caterer was selected. Everyone came except Vince's brother, who offered a "lame" excuse, according to Vince. Over the years, Vince's brother had made many attempts to reconcile, but Vince had remained adamant that the insult was too great to forgive. Eventually, Vince's brother had stopped offering apologies, since the rebuffs were always painful. As Vince grew closer to dying, he realized that he had lost twenty years of friendship with his brother because of an "unforgivable affront" that now seemed meaningless.

Vince's wife understood the pain her husband was experiencing and spent weeks convincing him to forgive his brother. With great trepidation, Vince called him and, during the ensuing conversation, was able to forgive him. It was a turning point in Vince's preparation for dying.

Asking for Forgiveness

Imagine knowing you did something that caused great pain to someone. Something that has haunted you your entire life. With effort, you were able to repress it, sometimes for years. But now, when you know you have little time left, it pops up like the mole in a carnival game: even if you can force the mole back into its hole, it just comes back up. Your loved one may wrestle with something like this that she feels can't be forgiven.

Twenty years before I met my patient Jean, she had abandoned her children and husband when her daughters were teenagers. Now, dying of emphysema, the only thing she wanted was her daughters' forgiveness. But even though they knew she was dying, they refused to see or talk to her. I suggested we write a forgiveness letter. Jean agreed on the condition that "they get it after I die." For three weeks, she dictated and I wrote. After many starts and stops, and numerous crumpled sheets of paper, we finally had something she felt good about. All her hard work was contained in two sentences: "Please forgive me. I've always loved you." It was enough to give her some peace before she died. Although it would have been better had her daughters come to her side to forgive her, what is ideal isn't always possible. If your loved one doesn't have the opportunity to ask for forgiveness directly from the person she believes she hurt, help her write a letter, or audio- or videotape her message.

Giving and Accepting Thanks

The dying have a need to thank those who have been important in their lives and in their dying. The usual responses to expressions of gratitude — "It was nothing" or "I enjoyed doing it" or "You don't need to thank me" — are socially appropriate in most situations. In our humbleness, we don't want to make more out of something than is necessary, especially if it took little effort on our part. But gratitude from someone who knows she is dying is so heartfelt that it needs to be accepted with graciousness and an understanding of what it means to the dying person. Thanks given to someone who has made that person's life wonderful, complete, or loving is not to be taken lightly. Understand that the dying person is telling you that you have been a central figure in her life, and that, without you, her life would have been less meaningful.

Thanking a dying loved one is just as profound. By thanking her for what she has done for you and others, you're saying she made a difference. A sense of satisfaction and peacefulness arises in a dying person when she can say, "I've done good. I've made a difference not only in what I have accomplished but also in what will continue on after I die."

Completing Mundane Things

Some people hold on to life despite pain in order to finish mundane things. Completing something that the dying person identifies as necessary can offer comfort as she approaches death. What she wants to complete may be only symbolic. One woman with multiple myeloma knew her condition was terminal. Whenever a dividend check arrived, she insisted that her daughter take it to the bank immediately. It was never an issue of needing the money. The checks were not substantial, and the assets of the woman were considerable. But she had an urgent need to leave nothing unfinished when she died. Start with the assumption that a similar insistence is related more to your loved one's state of mind than to any real urgency. Once you understand why your loved one may consider inconsequential things urgent, it becomes easier not to argue with her about the necessity of doing them.

ACTIVE DYING

Active dying signals that death is imminent. It could be hours or even days; predictions are rarely accurate. This stage can be identified by dramatic physical changes, such as a fixed gaze, lack of speech, graying of the skin, bluing of the skin under the fingernails and toe-nails, rapid breathing or pauses between inhalation and exhalation, a rattle when breathing, and dark urine or the absence of urine. A nurse will use changes in vital signs to confirm active dying. Some-times at the beginning of active dying, loved ones may slip in and out of consciousness.

What to Say and Not to Say

Since hearing is thought to be the last sense to stop, all conversa-tions in the presence of a dying loved one should be conducted with the assumption that she can hear you until the moment of death. This is a time to glorify the accomplishments and impact of your loved one. Let her know how important she has been in your life and the lives of others, and how her presence will continue in their accomplishments. This is a time to celebrate her life, not to mourn her death.

If your loved one has a history of welcoming touch, then touch her. One woman lay next to her husband and gently cradled him until he died. If your loved one was uncomfortable with physical contact, then simply holding her hand is appropriate. If you perceive in her a noticeable discomfort at being touched at this time, it's not a reflection on you. It is difficult to know what is happening physi-cally and psychologically as a person dies. And my suggestion here, as with everything else I've discussed in this book, is to allow her to let you know what she prefers.

During my last visit to one patient, I told her how much our short friendship had meant to me and how much I would miss her. She responded, "I've had a good life." She held on to my fingers tightly as she lost consciousness. When her daughter arrived thirty minutes later, she released my fingers.

The Vigil

A vigil is the time when we prepare for the imminent death of a loved one. If you haven't done it already, remove from the room as many items associated with a loved one's illness as you can and replace them with items, smells, and sounds associated with his life. If you feel uncomfortable at this time and you have hospice service, ask for a vigil volunteer. Many people feel discomfort when alone with someone at the moment of death, or when managing the friends and relatives who have gathered. Let the vigil volunteer handle everything. This person will come into your home, help create a calming environment, suggest things that can be done to ease the death of your loved one, and, if necessary, provide guidance to those who aren't sure what to do or who are causing your loved one discomfort.

Giving Permission to Die

How do you tell your loved one it's all right to die? Knowing what words you will use won't give you the slightest hint of what you'll feel when the words are said. The grief of some of my patients' family members was so consuming that it overshadowed the needs of their dying loved ones. They knew that death was imminent, but having these loved ones alive for even a few more hours or minutes was important to them. I never viewed their inability to let go as selfish. Rather, it was a conflict of interests. I've always felt that much of the reluctance to give a loved one permission to die has to do with the unfinished business of the caregiver.

What was so important that caregivers delayed their loved ones' departures, sometimes despite evidence of intense pain? The answer differed for each person, but usually it was something that had been left undone or unsaid. None of these things were so complicated that they couldn't have been addressed much earlier in the dying process. Just as loved ones need to complete their unfinished business to ease their deaths, so do caregivers, before the last moment, if they are to help their loved ones die.

THE MOMENT

Many poets and authors have tried to describe the sensations they feel at the moment of another person's death. Although I've been present at the deaths of others many times, I still can't find the words to describe that moment. When I do presentations, I ask if anyone has been present at the moment of someone's death; those who have, I ask what they experienced. Nobody felt they could put into words their emotions. Many spoke about a sense of spirituality that pervaded the room, their heightened sense of awareness, the flood of memories that surfaced, and an indescribable love for the person who just left. Nobody ever spoke about anything frightening; they described the actual moment of death as profoundly moving and always peaceful.

Choosing When to Die

Caregivers may decide to be with loved ones at the moment of death. The daughter of one patient stayed at her mother's side constantly once the latter entered active dying, talking to her and tending to her needs for two days. During the third day, she decided to leave for a few minutes to bring back some food. During the ten minutes of her absence, her mother died while those who served her in the hospice caressed her hands. When the daughter returned, she was crushed. "I shouldn't have left her side. What a horrible thing I did to her." We explained that it's not uncommon for a loved one to let go during the minutes when a caregiver leaves the room. One could argue that it's just coincidence. However, the number of times it occurs makes me think that dying may involve some volition. It's been argued that waiting for a caregiver to leave is a loved one's last gift, so that the caregiver doesn't experience the pain of watching a loved one die.

Conversely, some loved ones prolong their deaths until someone is at their side. When my brother-in-law was dying, my wife and daughter were at his side. A month before he went into active dying, I had promised him that I would be there to help him. When I heard his breathing pattern over the phone, my son and I took the next available plane from San Francisco to his East Coast home. During our stopover in Dallas, I called the apartment, and judging by the words of my daughter and wife, and by my brother-in-law's breathing pattern, I knew his death was imminent. I asked that the telephone be placed next to his ear, and I told him that we were on our way, but that if he felt he couldn't stay until we arrived, I would explain to my daughter and wife what they could do to make his passing easier. I knew he understood, because my daughter said a tear appeared. We did arrive before he died, and with all of us at his side he peacefully died.

Reside in the Spirituality of the Experience

After the moment of death, sit and do nothing. This is a time for caregivers and others who are present to reflect on what a loved one's life and death meant to them. During this time, preparation for grieving ends and healing begins. Shortly after one of my patients died at the hospice, I found his sister and brother-in-law at his side. They had been with him for a few hours.

"I don't think I've seen Bruce this peaceful since I met him," I said, after introducing myself.

"He really was an ornery curmudgeon," his sister said, "but we all loved him." She turned to her husband and said, "You remember that party we gave for him and Helen, don't you?" Her husband laughed and looked at his brother-in-law as if expecting him to comment.

"Yes, by the end of the party he'd managed to insult every single person, including the minister."

We spent the next hour talking about Bruce and his life. "Wasn't that true, Bruce?" his sister would say to him after relating a particularly funny story. Our interactions were neither solemn nor grieving. Rather, our celebration of Bruce's life created lasting memories for the three of us.

Rituals

It's easy to dismiss rituals as just the historical trappings of ancient religions, as something very beautiful but having little relevance to our contemporary lives. Nothing could be further from the truth. When Pope John Paul II died in 2005, Cardinal Theodore McCarrick of Washington, D.C., was asked by a newspaper reporter to comment on the various rituals that would be used for the funeral. The cardinal said that many of them were created during a period when most people weren't able to read. This explains their importance during medieval times. But how do you explain the power of ritual to begin healing in current times? Is there something so fundamental that it crosses all religious and nonreligious lines to reduce the grief we feel following the loss of a loved one? Ritual serves two important psychological functions. The first is to give us a connection to the past. Poet Robert Penn Warren says that history cannot give us a program for the future, but it can give us a fuller understanding of ourselves and our past.

Ritual can involve supplication through the act of kneeling for Catholics, through touching one's head to the ground for Muslims, and through prostrating for Buddhists. But it is not inherently related to religion. In my case, an improvised piece I played on my *shakuhachi* following the death of a patient fulfilled the role of ritual. In its second psychological function, ritual begins developing closure, as it did for a woman celebrating the passing of her best friend.

A traditional Irish wake was held, in which she surrounded her friend with flowers, incense, and pictures of their life together. The woman, along with other friends who attended the wake, remembered the wonderful times she'd had with her now-departed friend. Ritual is an important psychological event that connects us with the past and grounds us in the present.

Many people have found that cleaning the person's body in preparation for removal shows great respect and is also a healing ritual for everyone who participates. When my brother-in-law was dying, my wife, son, daughter, his favorite professional caregiver, and I surrounded him. Following his death, I asked everyone if they wished to participate in cleaning his body and preparing him for the mortician. Everyone agreed, but I could tell there was some discomfort. That quickly faded as we gently removed his bedclothes and washed his body with warm scented water. My wife focused on cleaning his face as everyone else ritually cleaned his body. As we did, each of us spoke about the impact he had made on us, and we retold touching stories about him. Once his body had been cleaned, we had to decide how we would dress him. We all agreed that he should leave us wearing his favorite T-shirt and shorts.

It's been three years since his death, and the image of my brother-in-law lying peacefully in bed wearing his favorite clothes still offers me comfort and a lasting memory of who he was and what he meant to us. Don't be afraid to invent your own ritual. The manner of preparation and the care taken will develop permanent touchstones for reducing your grief.

Contacting the Hospice or Mortuary

A medical person must officially pronounce the death of your loved one. There is a mistaken belief that someone has to be called immediately. Take your time. This is a very special moment you are having, and there is no legal or medical reason to cut it short. Call the hospice and let someone know your loved one has died and how much time you will need before the body can be removed. A hospice nurse will be sent. If you're not using a hospice and don't have a relationship with the mortician, delay the call. You'll know when you're ready to say good-bye. One final suggestion: remain present as the body is prepared for departure. Although it is a rare mortician who will handle a body with anything less than respect, being present will add to your peace of mind. At one of the hospices where I volunteered, it was a tradition to remain with the individual's body until it was removed from the house. It was always an honor to be chosen to fill that position.

FINAL THOUGHTS

Many people who have never witnessed a death imagine a Hollywood-style scene in which their loved one utters a quotable saying with her last breath, or a dramatic battle raging between the harbinger of death and the angels of heaven above the body of their loved one. In fact, witnessing your loved one's death will be the most spiritual event you'll ever experience — other than your own.

Preparing for death is a time for everyone to let go. And if you've understood what's necessary to help create the "good death," you and your loved one are ready. Of course you will grieve; it's difficult saying good-bye to someone who has been a part of your life and influenced it, and it's never easy giving up a part of your soul. But instead of displaying your grief to your loved one, it's a time to celebrate what you and the world gained by the way that he or she lived. It's like having an Irish wake, but with your loved one there to enjoy it.

We often remember things according to the impact they make on us. If you grieve excessively and focus on the soon-to-occur loss of your loved one, that will be the memory that stays with you. But celebrate that person's life by acknowledging what he or she contributed to yours, and your appreciation of your loved one's contributions will be what you remember. Without death, we wouldn't understand how precious life is, or understand why we should do the "right" thing every day we are alive. In gloriously saying good-bye to a precious soul, we help create a joyous death and — to slightly modify what Shakespeare said in *The Merchant of Venice* — we bless he who gives, and he who receives.

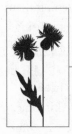

CHAPTER 7

Putting It All Together

Caregivers struggle to find a balance between meeting their loved ones' needs and meeting their own. Often that balance may involve painful choices, including giving up an exciting world filled with professional accolades for one that is isolating and not as rewarding. Or it may entail placing more importance on preserving a family's structure, and your own sanity, than on the wishes of a loved one. But many of the awful choices that caregivers believe they must make can be avoided by approaching caregiving differently. Try looking at the relationship between the caregiver and the loved one as mutually rewarding.

Caregiving is a way of learning something about yourself that may be impossible to discover through any other activity. Becoming responsible for someone's life and preparing him for a protracted illness or his death is transformative. You will come away from it with experiences that will change your life, knowing that you eased your loved one's death and voiced feelings and did things that will reduce the severity and duration of your own grieving.

Caregiving is unique, and few experiences prepare you for it. While many think caring for an infant is similar, infant care is an experience characterized more by love than by the conflicting emotions that pervade the care of an adult. But once you begin caring for an adult, what had appeared to be a daunting task becomes normal. Cleaning a loved one's body becomes no more frightening than washing a crystal glass, listening to his or her fear of death brings out in you the same compassion you once showed to a child afraid of a new experience, and remaining silent and supportive in the presence of agonizing pain becomes as natural as comforting a friend.

Lives and explanations that you have always evaluated in black and white terms, as right or wrong, correct or incorrect, become malleable, not through expediency, but because you have come to understand that the world works very differently at street level than when viewed through theories or doctrines.

The space occupied by the caregiver and loved one is special. Some would say spiritual. Depending on another person for one's continued existence creates a connectiveness unmatched in almost any other setting. The loved one is saying, "I can no longer continue living without your help." The caregiver's response is: "I'm honored by the opportunity to make the last phase of your life peaceful." When you accept that honor, you accept change. Change is inevitable in virtually all caregiving situations. It becomes a daily exercise in evolving to meet your loved one's needs. And while some of the experiences are enlightening, others can be unpleasant if taken at face value. Anger is just anger unless it is recognized as an expression of helplessness. Answering the same question many times is frustrating unless you recognize the questions as attempts to structure a world that is crumbling.

Caregiving is more a compassionate art than a science learned via lectures or books — even this one. The specifics of caregiving — or as I identify them in this book, my "suggestions" — are only guidelines. It's easy to explain why it's important to give someone permission to leave. But nobody can tell you exactly what you will feel as you say the words.

I can tell you this, though: You will soar to the heights of elation when you realize the enormous gifts you are giving your loved one and the gifts your loved one is giving you. You will also experience feelings so guilt-ridden that you'll never want to reveal them to another person. But living with contradictions, without judging them as either "good" or "bad," is a normal part of caregiving. Instead of pushing away those feelings, bring them closer and accept their legitimacy. Many of the problems in caregiving — for both caregiver and loved one — occur when the groundwork for the experience is ignored, and when crises are not anticipated but are dealt with at the moment they occur. A crisis state can be avoided by doing simple things in advance, such as accepting the legitimacy of all nonharmful requests.

Prepare for your loved one's future *now*, even if it seems time-consuming or pointless. And even if you have no intention of ever placing your loved one in a care facility, spend some time investigating such facilities. We never know what tomorrow or next week will bring. By doing things now, you can avoid some painful decisions.

Caregiving is not about magnificent gestures. It's about doing small, routine, and often time-consuming things, actions that say to your loved one: "I'm here for you, regardless of what you need." Your future and the future of your loved one will be shaped by what you do during the course of your caregiving. Following the suggestions in this book will help you avoid the regrets that other caregivers have experienced because they postponed their preparations until it was too late. We can't avoid the grief we will feel at the loss of a loved one. But we can avoid the grief of regretting that we left things unsaid or undone.

There is nothing objective about the world of caregiving. It takes place not in a laboratory under controlled circumstances but in a messy world where what we see is shaped by our beliefs, needs, and fears. And although many commonalities exist between the world of a caregiver and that of a loved one, some of the experiences of each are open to interpretation. A loved one may look at Claude Monet's *Impression, Sunrise* and see the most serene scene she could ever imagine. A caregiver may look at the same painting and see hazy images. A caregiver may think about bathing a loved one and know it will result in sore muscles from lifting. A loved one will anticipate the comfort of being clean. A caregiver looks at the world through the eyes of someone who has chosen to give up parts of his identity to serve another human being. A loved one looks at a world of few choices. In the dissimilar worlds of loved ones and caregivers are potholed roads that can be partially repaired, but usually not brought back to their pre-illness condition.

A number of years ago at a workshop, the Tibetan Buddhist monk Sogyal Rinpoche related a conversation that a counselor had had with a dying patient. The patient said he didn't need to have anyone understand what he was going through; that wasn't possible. But he wanted others to *act* as if they understood what he was going through. We may get close to understanding what loved ones go through, but I doubt we can ever *really* know. We can, however, be compassionate and try to understand the unskillful words and actions of loved ones as they attempt to express feelings that can no longer be communicated in traditional ways. Then anger will no longer be anger. Ingratitude will no longer be ingratitude. Both labels are distortions of what a loved one feels but can no longer express skillfully. The needs of loved ones and caregivers may be substantially different and, unfortunately, conveyed in unskillful ways. A caregiver may perceive criticism by a loved one, who is wrestling with the unfinished business of her life, as ingratitude rather than as the cry for help that it is. And doing so will lay the groundwork for pulling away from this loved one and inadvertently ignoring her legitimate needs.

The communicative ability of a loved one may decrease as an illness progresses. Some of the changes, such as the inability to retrieve words, may be immediately detectable. Others, such as not picking up satire or humor in a story, may be subtler. The ability to communicate and understand is a central feature of being human, and when it deteriorates so does the connection of a loved one to the world.

The more a caregiver can adjust to her loved one's changing abilities and simplify communication, the longer he will feel connected to the world.

As language slowly dissolves, so does a loved one's sense of organization. In many ways, language forms the connective tissue of our lives, structuring our experiences and thoughts. Seemingly bizarre or unskillful comments or behaviors are rarely directed at the people they end up hurting. When people are frightened or confused, their words and behaviors reflect their helplessness and hopelessness. As their ability to impose structure on the world deteriorates, we can offer external strategies to help them regain a sense of structure, such as calendars marked with events, and posters showing where family members are living.

Nothing lasts forever — neither the lives of our loved ones nor the sacrifices we make to care for them. At some point, you may become a kind of midwife for your loved one. Just as a midwife gently helps a newborn into the world, you can gently aid your loved one's passage at the other end of the continuum. Life departs in an orderly fashion. Sometimes it's quick, and at other times it lingers. Regardless of its speed, you are there to ease it along by minimizing whatever may interfere with its natural progression, and by maximizing whatever acts as a lubricant.

The death of a loved one will be painful for you, but it will also allow you to put into perspective the effect your loved one had on you and the world. Then, having completed one journey, you will be poised to start another. It's analogous to sitting on the edge of a dance floor and watching the dancers whirl to the rhythm of the music — so joyfully that they risk the embarrassment of tripping over their feet. You're invited to dance. Your impulse may be to politely decline, fearing you'll never be able to rejoin the living. But you can also say "Yes," realizing that stumbling is not such a bad thing, given what you can gain by accepting the invitation to dance.

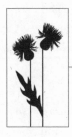

APPENDIX I

National and International Organizations

AIDS

AIDS Healthcare Foundation. This global organization provides cutting-edge medicine and advocacy to over one hundred thousand people in twenty-two countries. See www.aidshealth.org.

ALZHEIMER'S AND DEMENTIA

Alzheimer's Foundation. The world's leading voluntary health organization in Alzheimer's care, support, and research. See www.alz.org.

Alzheimer's Foundation of America. The goal of this organization is to provide optimal care and services to individuals confronting dementia, and to their caregivers and families, through member organizations dedicated to improving the quality of life. See www.alzfdn.org.

Huntington's Disease Society of America. The organization's goal is to fight Huntington's disease and improve the lives of people with this disease and of their families. See www.hdsa.org.

Lewy Body Dementia Association. Dedicated to raising awareness of the Lewy body dementias; supporting patients, their families, and caregivers; and promoting scientific advances. See www.lbda.org.

ARTHRITIS

Arthritis Foundation. A not-for-profit organization that addresses the more than one hundred types of arthritis and related conditions. See www.arthritis.org.

CANCER

American Cancer Society. A nationwide, community-based voluntary health organization, it is dedicated to eliminating cancer as a major health problem. See www.cancer.org.

Christians Overcoming Cancer. The organization provides awareness, emotional support, and financial relief services to cancer patients in active treatment. See www.christiansovercomingcancer.com.

Leukemia and Lymphoma Society. The society's goal is to promote the cure of leukemia, lymphoma, Hodgkin's disease, and myeloma and to improve the quality of life of patients and their families. See www.lls.org.

LIVESTRONG. This organization provides free, confidential, one-on-one support and resources to anyone affected by cancer, including those who have cancer, loved ones, caregivers, friends, and health care professionals. See www.livestrong.org.

Lotus Survival Foundation. This organization provides education and access to resources meant to assist those who have been affected by, or are concerned about, breast cancer. See www.lotussurvival foundation.org.

National Cancer Institute. Part of the National Institutes of Health, this institute is the federal government's principal agency for cancer research and training. See www.cancer.gov.

Prostate Cancer Foundation. This is a philanthropic source of support for prostate cancer research engaged in the effort to discover better treatments and a cure for prostate cancer. See www.pcf.org.

Susan G. Komen for the Cure (breast cancer). The organization is a global leader of the breast cancer movement, with a grassroots network of breast cancer survivors and activists working together to save lives, empower people, ensure quality care for all, and energize science to find the cures. See http://ww5.komen.org.

Us TOO International Prostate Cancer Education and Support Network. A grassroots network of 325 support groups worldwide, providing men and their families with free information, materials, and peer-to-peer support so they can make informed choices on detection, treatment options, and coping with ongoing survivorship. See www.ustoo.org.

CARDIOVASCULAR

American Heart Association. The mission of this national voluntary health agency is to reduce disability and death from cardiovascular diseases and stroke. See www.heart.org.

National Stroke Association. The goal of this association is to reduce the incidence and impact of stroke by developing compelling education programs and programs focused on prevention, treatment, rehabilitation, and support. See www.stroke.org.

DIABETES

American Diabetes Association. This association's purpose is to prevent and cure diabetes and to improve the lives of all people affected by diabetes. See www.diabetes.org.

LIVER

American Liver Foundation. The foundation facilitates, advocates, and promotes education, support, and research for the prevention, treatment, and cure of liver disease. See www.liverfoundation.org.

MUSCULAR

ALS Association. This association leads the way in global research, providing assistance for people with ALS through a nationwide network of chapters, coordinating multidisciplinary care through certified clinical care centers, and fostering government partnerships. See www.alsa.org.

Muscular Dystrophy Association. This nonprofit health agency is dedicated to curing muscular dystrophy, ALS, and related diseases by funding worldwide research. See www.mda.org.

National Multiple Sclerosis Society. The organization addresses the challenges of living with multiple sclerosis, funds research, drives change through advocacy, educates, and provides programs and services. See www.nationalmssociety.org.

PULMONARY

American Asthma Foundation. The only national organization funding research into the causes of asthma, which affects more than 24 million Americans. See www.americanasthmafoundation.org.

Chronic Obstructive Pulmonary Disease Foundation. This organization helps increase awareness about COPD, its management, and resources available to individuals with COPD and their caregivers. See www.copdfoundation.org.

MesotheliomaTreatment.net. This organization is an online resource for locating mesothelioma news, asbestos facts, and treatment options. See www.mesotheliomatreatment.net.

RENAL FAILURE

American Kidney Fund. The goal of this organization is to fight kidney disease through direct financial support to patients in need and by funding health education and prevention efforts. See www.akfinc.org.

National Kidney Foundation. This foundation is dedicated to preventing kidney and urinary tract diseases and improving the health and well-being of individuals and families affected by kidney disease. See www.kidney.org.

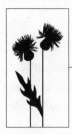

APPENDIX 2

Support Groups and Services

The following is only a partial listing of support groups found on Yahoo! and Facebook. With the exception of Memory People (on Facebook), all groups are listed on Yahoo! The descriptions are supplied by the groups.

ABI News 2U. Informs, educates, and enlightens others about TBI (traumatic brain injury) or ABI (acquired brain injury) and other subjects that we may want to tell others about. Archived newsletters have survivors' stories, articles, and links to provide other benefits for survivors and caregivers.

Advanced Prostate Cancer. Advanced prostate cancer and recurrent prostate cancer. Treatment information and support for men with prostate cancer that did not respond adequately to primary treatment. Rising posttreatment PSAs. Also for family, friends, and caregivers. Sponsored and produced by the national nonprofit prostate cancer organization Malecare.

Alzheimer's Disease Support and Information Group. We provide support and compassion to caregivers, friends, and patients dealing with

Alzheimer's disease and related or undiagnosed forms of memory problems or dementia.

Brain Tumor Treatments. This group is for patients/caregivers/doctors to discuss issues dealing with the treatment of brain tumors (brain cancer), including glioblastoma multiforme (GBM), anaplastic astrocytomas (AA), oligodendroglioma, brain mets, low-grade gliomas, and others.

Caregiver. Information, ideas, viewpoints, experiences, questions, suggestions, and comments on caring for the dependent adult.

Caregiver Connect. An online community for caregivers to share caregiving tips and support.

Care Givers Unite. A place for caregivers of loved ones to vent, share experiences, and support one another during this trying time in their and their loved ones' lives.

COPD Connect. Your connection to everything related to COPD and other pulmonary diseases. A support and information group for patients, caregivers, and professionals.

Coping Skill. Developing coping skills with: depression, anxiety, avoidant behavior (AvPD), social anorexia, voices-hearing (VH) schizophrenia (SZ), bipolar (BP), post–traumatic stress disorders (PTSD), multiple personality disorders (MPD, DID), stress disorder, panic attacks, agoraphobia, schizoid, and other disorders.

Elderly Parents. This group is for anyone who is caring for or has elderly parents (seniors), whether you're living with your parents, or living separately and caring for their needs, and whether they're sickly or healthy but need regular help.

Empowering Caregivers. A monthly newsletter that features expert columns, articles on caregiving, journal exercises, important news information, care-site- and caregiver-of-the-month spotlight, inspiration, humor, and more, while providing emotional and spiritual support. It is about choices, healing, and opening to love, the greatest healing power of all.

HD Caregivers. Designed to be a safe haven for those caring for someone with Huntington's disease. Members are encouraged to honestly express their feelings and situations with others who have "been there and done that," as well as with those who are anticipating similar situations. The goal is to provide a positive supportive environment.

Huntington's Disease Support Club. This support group is for everyone connected to Huntington's disease: those affected, tested positive, at-risk, tested negative, caregivers, family members, and friends. Our goal as a club is to offer support through unity and to work together to raise awareness and fun.

LBD Caregivers. An online support and information group for people whose loved ones suffer from Lewy body dementia.

Living with ALS. An avenue for persons living with ALS, and for their caregivers, to communicate with the ALS community immediately, to share information, ideas, support, and fellowship.

Memory People. A closed Facebook Group. You must have a Facebook account and ask to join. It's for all those with Alzheimer's, their caregivers, and advocates.

MSers Online. This list was created for anyone who has multiple sclerosis (MS), family members, relatives, caregivers, friends, and coworkers, and for you if you know someone who has been stricken with MS that you would like to help. You can provide support, advice, share common experiences, meet new friends, and discuss anything that deals with MS.

Open to Hope Foundation. An online resource center for people who have experienced loss. Our vision is that all people who experience loss will learn to live with their grief, cope with their pain, and invest in their future.

Senior Caregivers. This group is for those who are responsible for the care of senior members of their family or other elderly persons, a place for support for, advice for, and social interaction of such caregivers. All who provide this service to a loved one are invited to ask questions, provide answers, and share their experiences with the group.

Stroke Caregivers Support. This is a support list for stroke caregivers. If you are providing care and support to a parent, spouse, friend, or child who has had a stroke, please join us. We will listen, support, help, advise, and provide a sounding board for anyone dealing with stroke.

Stroke Survivors. We are primarily an online, international stroke support group for stroke survivors, caregivers, their families and friends, and interested health providers. Our group is a place to exchange our stories and information with others like ourselves, who are recovering from stroke or caring for strokers.

TBI Together. This list is where both survivors of TBI (traumatic brain injury) and caregivers can come together to learn from each other's perspectives. It is hoped that both groups will take time to read and "listen" to the opinions expressed; please do respect the fact that all here have loss, all need support to grow and learn to care.

The Pancreatitis Place. This group gives those whose lives are affected by pancreatic disorders, such as chronic pancreatitis or SOD, a safe, open environment to learn and share. In this caring environment, members discuss such things as treatments, procedures, pain, getting diagnosed, causes, diabetes, and disability, to name a few aspects of pancreatic disorders.

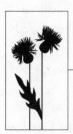

APPENDIX 3

Governmental Agencies

Administration on Aging. Designed to develop a comprehensive, coordinated, and cost-effective system of home- and community-based services that help elderly individuals maintain their health and independence in their homes and communities. See www.aoa.gov.

Caregivers Resources. Here you can find a nursing home, assisted living facility, or hospice; check your eligibility for benefits; get resources for long-distance caregiving; review legal issues; and find support for caregivers. See www.usa.gov/Citizen/Topics/Health /caregivers.shtml.

Disability. Provides an interactive, community-driven information network that focuses on disability-related programs, services, laws, and benefits. See https://www.disability.gov.

Medicare Comprehensive Links. Over 1 million people identified as eligible for this benefit are apparently not aware of this fact. For information regarding Medicare, call 800-333-7586, or visit the Medicare website at www.medicare.gov.

National Family Caregiver Support Program. Available throughout the United States. You can contact the program through a local Area Agency on Aging or by calling the Administration on Aging directly at 202-619-0724. There is no charge for any of the services provided to family caregivers of older persons. See www.agingcarefl.org/care giver/NationalSupport.

Social Security Administration. For information about Social Security disability benefits, the Supplemental Security Income program, or Medicare, call the U.S. Social Security Administration toll-free at 800-772-1213. The Social Security website is www.ssa.gov.

Veterans Administration Health Care. Use the main link for navigating to any services that are offered. See www.va.gov.

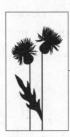

APPENDIX 4

End-of-Life Forms

MEDICAL CARE POWER OF ATTORNEY

Legal Help Mate. Medical Care Power of Attorney forms for each state are offered here for a fee. See www.legalhelpmate.com/poa.

Mayo Clinic. This website offers an explanation of the Medical Care Power of Attorney and what it should cover. See www.mayoclinic .com/health/living-wills/HA00014.

Nolo Law for All. This website, too, offers an explanation of the Medical Care Power of Attorney and what it should cover. See www.nolo.com.

DO NOT RESUSCITATE (DNR)

California Medical Association. For a small fee, this association supplies copies of the state's DNR form; the form may need to be modified for use in other states. See www.cmanet.org/resource-library /detail.dT?item=do-not-resuscitate-dnr-form-english.

Medline Plus. This healthcare information website explains the elements of a DNR. See www.nlm.nih.gov/medlineplus/ency/article /001908.htm.

Merck. The Merck drug company explains the ethical and legal issues involved in a DNR document. See www.merckmanuals.com/home /fundamentals/legal_and_ethical_issues/do-not-resuscitate_dnr _orders.html?qt=&sc=&alt=.

LIVING WILL

AllLaw.com. This website provides an explanation of the Living Will. See www.alllaw.com/articles/wills_and_trusts/article7.asp.

DoYourOwnWill.com. Provides a free Living Will form that can be adapted for use in any state. See www.doyourownwill.com/living -will/states.html.

Living Will U.S. Registry. A fee-based service that stores Living Wills and makes them computer accessible. See www.uslivingwillregistry .com.

FIVE WISHES

Aging with Dignity. Explains the document and supplies a low-cost form. See www.agingwithdignity.org.

PHYSICIAN ORDERS FOR LIFE-SUSTAINING TREATMENT (POLST)

Coalition for Compassionate Care. Information and forms are available here. See www.coalitionccc.org.

National POLST Paradigm Task Force. The site offers information and forms. See www.ohsu.edu/polst.

CONSERVATORSHIP

Wikipedia. Provides the legal definition of conservatorship. See http://en.wikipedia.org/wiki/Conservatorship.

GUARDIANSHIP

Chiff.com. Provides the legal definition of guardianship. See www.chiff.com/legal/elder-law.htm.

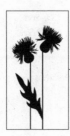

Index

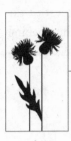

About the Author

Stan Goldberg, PhD, was named the Hospice Volunteer Association's Volunteer of the Year in 2009. His book *Lessons for the Living* won the London Book Festival's Grand Prize for Best New International Book of 2009 and was featured in *The Best Buddhist Writing 2010*. A hospice bedside and vigil (period of active dying) volunteer for many years, he has served more than four hundred patients and their loved ones at four different hospices, and was also a trainer and consultant at each. As a professor of communicative disorders at San Francisco State University and a private therapist, he counseled clients and did research on how to understand and communicate difficult emotions. Over a period of thirty years, he taught more than three thousand graduate students in speech-language pathology to implement techniques based on his original research.

He was a bedside volunteer at the internationally known Zen Hospice Project in San Francisco for two years, until its Guest House closed. Subsequently, he had similar responsibilities with Hospice By The Bay, the second-oldest home hospice agency in the country, and the George Mark Children's House, the first free-standing hospice for children in the United States. He currently serves as a bedside volunteer at Pathways Home Healthcare and Hospice, in the San

Francisco Bay Area, and is involved in that organization's volunteer training and philanthropy programs. He was a special guest of the South Korean government's National Cancer Center at the opening of its Proton Beam Therapy Center. He lives in San Francisco, California. His website is stangoldbergwriter.com.

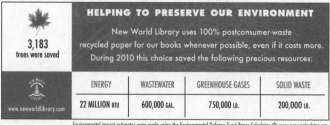

HELPING TO PRESERVE OUR ENVIRONMENT

3,183 trees were saved

New World Library uses 100% postconsumer-waste recycled paper for our books whenever possible, even if it costs more. During 2010 this choice saved the following precious resources:

ENERGY	WASTEWATER	GREENHOUSE GASES	SOLID WASTE
22 MILLION BTU	600,000 GAL.	750,000 LB.	200,000 LB.

Environmental impact estimates were made using the Environmental Defense Fund Paper Calculator @ www.papercalculator.org.